Healthcare, Guaranteed

Healthcare, Guaranteed

A Simple, Secure Solution for America

Ezekiel J. Emanuel, M.D., Ph.D

with a Foreword by Victor R. Fuchs, Ph. D

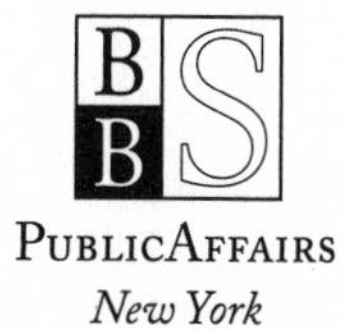

PublicAffairs
New York

Published in the United States by PublicAffairs™,
a member of the Perseus Books Group.

Printed in the United States of America.

Library of Congress Cataloging-in-Publication Data
Emanuel, Ezekiel J., 1957-
Healthcare, guaranteed : a simple, secure solution for America / Ezekiel J. Emanuel ; with a foreword by Victor R. Fuchs. — 1st ed.
p. ; cm.
Includes bibliographical references and index.
ISBN 978-1-58648-662-4 (pbk.)
1. Medical care—United States. 2. Health care reform—United States. 3. Insurance, Health—United States. I. Title.
[DNLM: 1. Insurance, Health—United States. 2. Delivery of Health Care—economics—United States. 3. Health Care Reform—United States. 4. Universal Coverage—United States. W 275 AA1 E495 2008

RA395.A3E43 2008
362.1'04250973—dc22

2008007746

First Edition

10 9 8 7 6 5 4 3 2 1

To

Rebekah,

Gabrielle,

and

Natalia

Whose commitments to

social justice inspire me.

CONTENTS

The views expressed in this book are Dr. Emanuel's and do not represent the official views or policies of the Department of Health and Human Services, The National Institutes of Health, or the Public Health Service. This book was undertaken as an outside activity separate from Dr. Emanuel's official NIH duties.

FOREWORD

by Victor R. Fuchs

Does America need another new book on health policy? Yes, it does—for three important reasons.

First, other books that describe the shortcomings of American healthcare—unrelenting hikes in cost, almost 50 million uninsured, dangerous lapses in quality, and more—usually blame insurance companies, drug manufacturers, organized medicine, or some other convenient scapegoat. Such criticism, while sometimes justified, does not get to the heart of the problem. The system itself is dysfunctional. No doubt there are some organizations and individuals that lack integrity or competence, but this book shows that the major shortcomings of American healthcare are the result of deep and irreparable flaws in the way the country finances, organizes, and delivers care.

Second, many books offer partial cures for reducing the number of uninsured or reducing costs, but these incremental changes provide only temporary relief, at best. Problems of access, cost, and quality are related; they must be tackled simultaneously through a coordinated approach. This book makes the case that only comprehensive reform can heal our ailing healthcare system—and keep it healthy.

Finally, this book provides the reader with a clear picture of a coordinated approach—one based on universal healthcare vouchers. It identifies the essential elements for making the nation's healthcare more equitable and more efficient in a manner congruent with basic American values. It also specifies the conditions that might make such reform a reality.

EZEKIEL EMANUEL AND I collaborated on the development of a universal voucher approach and described it in outline form in the *New York Times* (November 18, 2003), somewhat more fully in *The New England Journal of Medicine* (March 24, 2005), and more fully still in a Brookings Institution Hamilton Project paper (July 2007). See Further Reading, Chapter Four. The advantages of such an approach over other reform proposals are numerous and, in my judgment, compelling.

According to this proposal **everyone** would receive insurance for basic healthcare. Coverage does not depend on income, employment status, health status, household living arrangements, or any other characteristic.

The cost of basic healthcare for all would be fairly determined by the individual's ability to pay. Everyone purchasing goods and services would bear their proportional share of healthcare costs.

Administrative costs, currently estimated between 15 and 25 percent of total costs, would be sharply reduced.

Insurance subsidies for the poor and the sick would be fairly and efficiently allocated. The implicit subsidies would adjust automatically with changes in income or health status.

Because funding for the proposed plan derives from a dedicated tax, the public's desire to increase benefits must be matched by its willingness and ability to pay with higher taxes. The experience of other countries shows that this is the only dependable way of controlling costs.

Elimination of employer health insurance substantially increases the efficiency of U.S. labor markets. Workers and employers will benefit and a major source of labor-management friction is eliminated.

The substitution of the Guaranteed Healthcare Access Plan for federal–state programs, such as Medicaid and S-CHIP, significantly reduces major financial and administrative burdens on state governments. Medicare would be replaced over time, without disrupting coverage of its current beneficiaries.

Last, but certainly not least, by funding an independent Institute for Technology and Outcomes Assessment and by guaranteeing patient choice among competing qualified health plans, the proposal outlined in this book sets the stage for improvements in quality and decreases in cost.

Patients, health professionals, government officials, employers, union leaders, taxpayers, and other concerned readers will gain valuable insight into the following questions:

- Why is the United States the only high-income country without universal health insurance?
- Why does the United States spend twice as much on healthcare as European countries, whose citizens live as long or longer than Americans?
- Why is there so much over-use, under-use, and misuse of medical technology?
- Why has healthcare coverage become the flashpoint for labor/management disputes and the primary cause of many costly strikes?
- Why does such a large percentage of the U.S. healthcare dollar go toward administration and marketing, duplication of services, and expensive interventions of little or no value to patients?

Some readers may wish that the book provided more details, but, in my judgment, it wisely refrains from doing so. Sometimes the "devil is in the details," but in order to blaze a path to sustainable, comprehensive reform, it is more important to recognize that "God is in the essentials." A reform plan that doesn't get the main points about funding, organization, and delivery right will not succeed regardless of how much the details are tweaked. Obsessing on details often turns out to be a strategy for blocking reform.

Other readers may wish there was more discussion of the politics of healthcare reform. Again, the author shows admirable restraint. There is no shortage of players on the political scene willing to pronounce about political feasibility, often as an indirect way of opposing change. In my experience, such pronouncements cost nothing to produce, and are usually worth about the same. American history is studded with examples of major social, economic, and political innovations that experts deemed to be "off the radar screen" only to be enacted some years later.

By the end of this book (it is a short one), the reader will have a clearer understanding of how America got into the current healthcare mess, the obstacles that stand in the way of a better system, and the essentials needed to solve the problems of high costs, uninsured individuals, quality lapses, and the unsustainable growth of healthcare expenditures.

VICTOR R. FUCHS
Henry J. Kaiser Jr. Professor Emeritus
Stanford University

CHAPTER 1

Beyond Anecdotes

The American healthcare system is a dysfunctional mess. In the United States, healthcare costs over $2,100,000,000,000—that's $2.1 *trillion*—per year, or more than one out every six dollars spent on everything in the entire United States. On an individual basis, the care tab comes to more than $7,000 per person. This is 50 percent higher per person than in second-place Switzerland and nearly double what neighboring Canada spends.

Yet despite these fantastic sums of money being spent, the health status of America's citizens looks sickly when measured against the tallies in other industrialized countries. Our infant mortality rate is twice as high as that of Japan, Sweden, and Norway, even among whites. We have lower life expectancy than the Japanese, French, Canadians, and Germans. Even among adults who reach age 60, Americans expect to live another 16.6 years while in other industrialized countries the average is another 19.1 years. Annually, we lose a higher percentage of lives to the ravages of diabetes than people in other developed nations, perhaps because, when compared to

Europeans and Australians, fewer Americans have a regular physician. Fewer American patients hospitalized with heart attacks or pneumonia receive recommended care than patients in other countries. And only 49 percent of Americans receive screening and preventive care compared to 80 percent in many other countries. Americans feel the impact in their wallets and in their lives. Skimpy health insurance, or lack of any coverage at all, is the main reason why more than half of patients cite "cost" as the reason they have failed to fill prescriptions or skipped tests and treatments. All other industrialized countries around the world provide quality care for every one of their citizens at a lower per capita cost than in the United States. If they can do it, certainly we Americans can.

Americans are frustrated and mystified. None of these factors—not the choices, the costs, or the scope of coverage—quite make sense. Graphic, tragic stories about America's healthcare system have become media staples. You know things have taken a downturn when Hollywood releases movies about the catastrophic state of American healthcare, and when the largest healthcare insurer, United Healthcare, takes out a full page ad in the *Wall Street Journal* (March 19, 2007) that declares "[t]he health system isn't healthy. There's no denying it. A system that was designed to make you feel better often just makes things worse."

Ominous declarations and heartbreaking stories in books like *Sick* and movies like *Sicko* are necessary to get Americans to acknowledge that there is an undeniable problem. But as distressing as these stories are, and as angry as people have become, solving the healthcare mess requires more than sharing sadness, shock, and frustration. We need to move beyond anecdotes to bridge the gap between the symptoms and the cure.

Any reform of our healthcare system, even one that is laid out in broad brush strokes, requires more than digestible narrative. And while policy talk alienates many smart, well-meaning citizens, there is no escaping the need for systematic policy analysis and discussion in strategizing how to change the system. As Euclid reminded Ptolemy I, the King of Egypt: "There is no royal road to geometry."

Even health policy experts and brilliant people are challenged to grapple with the ins-and-outs of a system comprising nearly 1 million acute hospital beds, 850,000 physicians, 2.5 million nurses, about 1,000 health insurance companies, and more than 3 billion prescriptions. The jargon—reinsurance; SNF; CPT codes; Medicare Parts A, B, C, and D; RBRVS; DME/IME; EMTALA; and MedPAC—along with the profusion of proposed reforms only add to the confusion. These complexities may be good sleeping aids, but they offer little help in getting anything positive accomplished.

This intricate web makes it so difficult to accurately predict how any proposed change will affect powerful stakeholders, much less individual families, that in the end it is less scary to stick with a system that is broken than to risk the repairs. Inevitably, the frustration from this inertia bubbles over into a blame game. Not so long ago, hard-hearted managed-care companies were the villains of healthcare. They were replaced by unscrupulous malpractice lawyers, greedy drug companies, and blood-sucking insurance companies. Who's next?

Everyone involved in the healthcare system is in some way at fault. Some, like HealthSouth, Tenet, Hospital Corporation of America (HCA), and TAP Pharmaceuticals, are guilty of fraud. Others, such as the pharmaceutical companies that charge $100,000 or more for a single drug, are preying on often-desperate patients eager for cures. Physicians who run Medicaid mills, perform unnecessary operations, or prescribe unnecessary treatments meddle with the system for their own rather than their patients' good. But seeking scapegoats tends to offer only unsatisfying simplistic solutions. A patient's bill of rights, electronic medical records, limits on malpractice claims for pain and suffering, re-importation of drugs from Canada or Mexico, wellness programs rather than a "healthcare system" for the sick—these, and more, have been offered up in response to flawed policies. And although they might contribute to a solution, none of these approaches constitutes a cure for the disarray we politely call a healthcare system.

For me, the broken healthcare system is personal.

My father is a pediatrician, and from him I absorbed the noble and heroic facets of medicine. The late nights rushing to a hospital to save a child, the free care given to families who could not afford doctor visits, and the campaigns to remove lead paint from apartments all served as my early education about the healthcare system. On weekends, my brothers and I used to accompany our father on hospital rounds, witnessing how he gently examined babies and talked to new mothers. Seeing my father's dedication as well as the tremendous gratitude from the families he cared for, and having a "good head" for science, meant I was bound for medicine at a young age.

In medical school, however, I began to experience the less ideal, more dysfunctional aspects of the healthcare system. My first day on the cancer ward, while rounding with a medical team, I met a teenager who was receiving chemotherapy for her Hodgkin's disease—a cancer of the immune system. She had been admitted for low blood counts, fever, and a suspected infection. Her platelets were low at 19,000 (typical levels are between 150,000 and 400,000), and the team ordered a transfusion. Not being the quiet and reserved type, I asked why they were ordering a transfusion. "We transfuse patients when their platelets drop below 20,000," went the explanation. "Why 20,000?" I asked, noting that some of my friends who were in medical school on the West Coast transfused platelets only when the platelets dropped below 10,000. "Are there any data showing that transfusing at 20,000 is better than transfusing at 10,000 or 5,000?" "That's what we do here," came the reply. This was my first, but far from last, lesson in how medical decisions are made, and how often they are made based on "what we do here" rather than on any hard research.

A few years later, I experienced one of the enormous frustrations of being an intern: caring for the patients we cruelly called "frequent flyers" when we were called in the middle of the night, dead-tired, to admit them. Typically, these were patients suffering from congestive heart failure or emphysema, who had been aggressively treated in the hospital, but returned just days after discharge with the same swollen legs or difficulty breathing that prompted their previous admission. We had worked hard to "tune them up," having them pee out their extra fluid or opening up their airways to ease their breathing problems. But when they walked out the door, there was no follow-up. No nurse called them or visited their home to weigh them, to encourage them to keep their legs up and to keep special stockings on, to prevent them from overeating and drinking, to make sure they were using their inhalers properly and taking their other medicines on schedule. When the fluid re-accumulated, they became short of breath and ended up, once again, in the emergency room. And the cycle started all over. We treated them aggressively, got them in good shape, and sent them home—only to see them back again in a few days or weeks. Because of our fragmented healthcare system, the hospital—the most expensive place to deliver medical care—had become the only place where care could be coordinated.

I decided to train as a breast oncologist, having been drawn to the field because it posed the most challenging issues in medicine. Cancer patients and their families face difficult life-and-death choices, treatments are extreme and extremely expensive, and trying experimental drugs is the norm. Getting to know struggling patients and families, and helping them navigate their way through such challenges, was an honor. Yet by the third month of training at the Dana-Farber Cancer Institute in Boston, I had become frustrated by the mindless routines. After I saw a patient, during which time we discussed the options and agreed on a treatment course, I would have to write up an informed-consent document by hand to tell the patient what the side effects of the drugs were. There was no template to follow, and what I wrote down about the side effects of the drugs was haphazard and varied from day to day; it frequently depended on which side effects came to mind because of what my patients were experiencing that day. I also found myself handwriting the orders for the right dosages of the chemotherapy drugs—the same three-drug combination for many of my breast cancer patients, the same two-drug combination for most of my colon cancer patients, and another multi-drug combination for my lung cancer patients. Spending hours a day repeatedly writing the same informed-consent forms and the same chemotherapy orders was, to say the least, tedious—certainly not what I had trained years and years to do. And, given my terrible doctor's handwriting, which only got more indecipherable the more—and faster—I had to write, it was not uncommon for the nurse or pharmacist to call me to "clarify" one of the orders. What if we had standard, preprinted informed-consent forms for each drug? And what if there were standard, preprinted pharmacy orders for the most common chemotherapy combinations? This would free me—and the other junior doctors—to spend more valuable time talking to and caring for patients. I proposed the idea to one of the senior doctors. It went nowhere.

Several years later, in 1994, tragedy struck the Dana-Farber. Betsy Lehman, a 39-year-old mother of two and a health reporter for the *Boston Globe*, was battling metastatic breast cancer. With her husband, himself a cancer researcher, she decided to undergo an experimental bone marrow transplant. Unfortunately, within days her heart failed and she died. No one could figure out why. Months later, an auditor decoded the pharmacy order sheet. The chemotherapy order was written incorrectly. Betsy Lehman had received a massive overdose of toxic drugs for four days. Fortunately, the Dana-Farber has worked hard in subsequent years to introduce electronic physician ordering, becoming a leader in implementing patient safety measures. But many hospitals have not yet learned the lesson.

It was also in the early 1990s that, frustrated, I took the lessons I was learning and began thinking more intensively about improving healthcare. I developed a general proposal for healthcare vouchers. After the 1992 presidential election, I served on President Clinton's Healthcare Task Force. President Clinton's Health Security Act was voted down in 1994.

From that failure, I learned a great deal about the many ways a well-meaning reform effort can go wrong. I learned not to design a reform so complex that few people can understand it. I learned how important it is to have a powerful group or set of groups that will champion and fight for the reform instead of distancing themselves when the going gets rough. Most importantly, I learned that we must be ready. The window of opportunity to enact a reform will be open only a short time. It is crucial that we not wait until after the electoral mandate to begin crafting the proposal. Rather, we need to have to have a well-thought-out and tested plan ready the next time the opportunity presents itself.

In 2003, I started working to more systematically develop my ideas on healthcare reform. I began collaborating with Victor Fuchs, who had his own reform plan. Vic is one of the original healthcare economists and, even more significant, one of the most original thinkers on healthcare in the United States. Over the last five years, we have worked together intensively to elaborate upon, refine, and test the reform proposal now called the Guaranteed Healthcare Access Plan. What are its essential elements?

First, it guarantees all Americans health coverage—and by *all* we mean 100 percent of them. Every American receives a healthcare certificate that covers his or her health insurance. The certificate covers a standard set of benefits, the same benefits that members of Congress now receive—office and home visits, hospitalization, preventive screening tests, prescription drugs, some dental care, inpatient and outpatient mental-health care, and physical and occupational therapy. This coverage is much more generous than Medicare's and better than the insurance that 85 percent of Americans get. And it will be totally portable. Insurance companies will have to cover everyone who brings them a certificate and will have to guarantee renewal each year. They will *not* be able to exclude anyone or deny payment for preexisting conditions. This will prevent them from cherry-picking only healthy people.

Private insurance companies or health systems will put together networks of doctors, hospitals, home healthcare agencies, and other providers to deliver care in a coordinated way.

Using their certificates, Americans will choose their health plan, their doctor, and their hospital. They will also be able to choose whether to buy a "platinum" plan at their own expense with additional services above the standard ones.

There will no longer be a need for employer-based health insurance. The Guaranteed Healthcare Access Plan will belong to the individual, ensuring complete portability. Workers will no longer have to fear losing coverage if they switch jobs, start their own company, or become unemployed. In addition, because employers will no longer pay for healthcare, the premiums won't come out of workers' paychecks. No one will be forced to leave Medicare, Medicaid, or other government programs, but there will also be no new enrollees. Over time, Medicare and Medicaid will be phased out. All Americans will get their coverage through the Guaranteed Healthcare Access Plan.

There will be a National Health Board with twelve Regional Boards to oversee and monitor the system. The Boards will regularly review the standard benefits covered, monitor the health plans, and oversee other workings of the system.

By ending employer-based insurance as well as government-provided health coverage, the Guaranteed Healthcare Access Plan will lower state and federal taxes. The Plan saves money by eliminating a lot of the insurance waste and bureaucratic red tape involved in determining who is eligible for various government programs. Also, no premiums will be deducted from workers' paychecks. Instead, the health certificates will be paid for by a dedicated value-added tax (VAT)—one that functions much like a sales tax. Being dedicated, funds will go only toward healthcare; they cannot be diverted to defense, Social Security, or any other program.

This way of paying for healthcare also provides credible cost control. We cannot spend more than the VAT brings in. If Americans want more healthcare services, they will have to lobby and convince Congress to increase the VAT. To further control healthcare costs, there will be an Institute for Technology Outcomes and Assessment. The Institute's responsibilities will include reviewing research studies and data on the effectiveness and cost of various drugs, devices, diagnostic tests, and new technologies—thus ensuring that we spend money only on those healthcare tests and treatments that truly improve the quality and length of life. To guarantee that the health plans don't skimp on care, the Institute will regularly collect and publish data from the health plans on how their patients are doing. And to solve the malpractice mess, there will be Centers for Patient Safety and Dispute Resolution to review complaints and compensate patients who are injured by medical error.

One of the real advantages of the Guaranteed Healthcare Access Plan is that it removes employers from the healthcare arena so they can focus on their core business. Businesses will decide whether to hire people based on their productivity, not on how much they will increase healthcare costs. The Plan will preempt labor-management conflict, which, over the last decade, has focused exclusively on healthcare costs. Over time, it should also increase employment and reduce the incentive for outsourcing. For workers, it will totally end job-lock and, with premiums no longer deducted from their paychecks, even increase their income.

Another great strength of the Guaranteed Healthcare Access Plan is that it coheres with core American values: individualism and equality of opportunity. It protects all Americans through a standard benefits package that is guaranteed, but individuals who want more healthcare can use their own money to buy it. The Guaranteed Healthcare Access Plan marries the advantages of the market with the advantages of government. It lets companies compete in the market and innovate with new mechanisms to deliver high-quality care efficiently, while ensuring that they are accountable through government oversight.

In 2007, when presidential candidates were considering what to do about healthcare, I was asked to participate in a debate about the various options for reform. One of my "opponents" was Jonathan Gruber, the MIT economist who developed Massachusetts' healthcare reform plan, advised Governor Schwarzenegger on his reform, and is the leading advocate of the mandate reform proposal (see Chapter 6). In that debate, Gruber acknowledged that the Guaranteed Healthcare Access Plan was the best policy proposal for healthcare. It was efficient, equitable, and sustainable. His only reservation was whether it was politically feasible. Could it be enacted?

Whenever I present the Guaranteed Healthcare Access Plan, many people agree with Gruber. They acknowledge that it is the best reform plan but worry whether the country is up for such a big change. It is a big mistake to limit our thinking based on what we imagine is politically feasible. For one thing, we are frequently wrong. And by thinking only inside the box, we are likely to be too cautious and miss important reforms and opportunities. The healthcare mess is a big problem, one that demands a comprehensive solution. We have been filling in the cracks for decades—an approach that will not solve the healthcare system's dysfunctions in a sustainable way. Most importantly, Americans are not afraid of confronting a challenge. When we put our minds to it, we can overcome seemingly insurmountable barriers. We cannot throw in the towel before we have even tried to do the right thing. To understand what the Guaranteed Healthcare Access Plan is and why it is the right solution, we must begin by thinking through what kind of healthcare system we want and why the current one is failing.

CHAPTER 2

The Goals of Reform

The American healthcare system is unique. It has been built up over time, often by accident, occasionally through conscious decisions about how we pay for care, how we deliver care, and how we organize care—or don't—that largely reflect American society from the turn of the twentieth century until the 1960s. But to fix what is broken will require a unique solution that not only embraces the uniquely American values of individualism and equality of opportunity but also reflects the high-tech American society of the twenty-first century.

What goals should a healthcare reform proposal meet? A new American healthcare system should guarantee coverage for all, control costs, and improve quality of care. While these three objectives are essential, they must also rest on a solid foundation. For example, "guaranteed coverage" is a goal everyone can agree on, but guaranteed coverage of what, exactly? If we are going to guarantee coverage that we can afford, we need to define a standard set of benefits for all Americans. And if we're going to control costs, we must also streamline the financing mechanism for healthcare. The current employer-based coverage and our mish-mash of government programs create many cracks for people to fall through and drain economic resources. Because everything in healthcare is interconnected, modernizing how we finance care is linked to the goal of modernizing the delivery system itself. In order to provide coordinated, high-quality healthcare, in place of the disjointed care we now receive, we need to change financial incentives and the way we pay for care. Although the public does not always realize it, today's doctors deliver evidence-based care only about half the time—a failing due not to lack of hard work and dedication but to far more fundamental problems with the financing and organization of care.

The new American healthcare system must not only guarantee coverage at a reasonable cost, it must also preserve choice. Our supermarket shelves bulge with choices. In the far more vital realm of healthcare, Americans clamor just as loudly for the chance to choose. We want to choose our insurance plans, our hospitals, our doctors, and the option to buy the platinum or titanium models beyond the standard services guaranteed in the new system.

Beyond choice, we also demand equity. When it comes to financing, Americans want a fair funding mechanism, one requiring that all citizens support the healthcare system according to their ability. A reasonable method for handling disputes must replace our malfunctioning malpractice system. Last but not least, a well-designed healthcare system must stimulate economic revitalization rather than drag down businesses and government agencies.

The seven goals discussed above are summarized in Table 2.1. Together, they define the vision for a new American healthcare system. I strongly believe that they are attainable and that attaining them will largely solve the critical problems associated with healthcare in the United States today. This is a big assertion, and many Americans might be skeptical. Here is why it will work.

TABLE 2.1. PROPOSED HEALTHCARE GOALS

GOALS, QUESTIONS, AND CHARACTERISTICS OF THE CURRENT SYSTEM*

1. Guaranteed Coverage

Does the proposal for a new American healthcare system guarantee healthcare coverage for all Americans—not 96 percent or 97 percent, but 100 percent? Does the proposal guarantee a defined set of benefits that includes office and home visits, hospitalization, preventive screening tests, prescription drugs, some dental care, mental-health care, and physical and occupational therapies, with no deductibles and minimal co-payments?

Forty-seven million Americans lack health insurance.

2. Effective Cost Controls

Does the proposal improve efficiency by reducing excessive administrative costs and reducing fraud? Does the proposal eliminate multiple

*Tables 2.1, 4.4, 5.1, 6.2, and 7.2 all display the same initial Goals and Questions. Only the Characteristics (or Answers) are different in each case. A Comparative Summary (consisting of the four Healthcare Systems—Guaranteed Healthcare Access, Incremental Reform, Mandates, and Single-Payer) is located at the end of Chapter 8.

financing mechanisms and redundant bureaucracies? Will the proposal rein in rising costs of healthcare inflation from diffusion of technology and cost-ineffective care?

Each year for the last three decades, healthcare costs, on average, have risen 2.1 percent faster than the economy. Employers typically pay 11 percent of premiums for insurance administration. Medicare and Medicaid have reported at least 10 percent fraud. Medicaid and SCHIP spend considerable funds for means testing to determine eligibility.

3. High-Quality, Coordinated Care

Does the reform proposal have a mechanism to reduce medical errors, hospital-acquired infections, and high-cost/low-to-no-benefit treatments? Does the proposal encourage coordinated care and innovation in delivery, while also holding providers accountable for high-quality health outcomes? Is there a process for regularly evaluating the quality of these providers?

The healthcare delivery system is a fragmented, fee-for-service arrangement that emphasizes delivering more services rather than the right services. There have been many cases of underuse of proven tests and treatments, overuse of unproven tests and treatments, as well as tens of thousands of deaths from preventable medical errors.

4. Choice

Will Americans be able to choose their health insurance plans, physicians, and hospitals? Does the proposal give citizens the freedom to purchase extra healthcare benefits beyond the standard benefits guaranteed to all?

Some Americans have a choice of doctors, hospitals, and insurance companies. But for most workers, their employer decides what their insurance company will be. Many people on Medicaid—and, in-

creasingly, Medicare—are being refused treatment because government payments are so low.

5. Fair Funding

Does the proposal have financing in which all Americans contribute fairly?

Because of tax laws, the rich pay less for employer-based health insurance than the poor, and many working people do not have health insurance from their employers but earn too much to get Medicaid, which they support through their taxes.

6. Reasonable Dispute Resolution

Does the new healthcare system proposal offer a mechanism for rational dispute resolution that quickly and efficiently compensates patients who are harmed while at the same time protecting physicians from frivolous lawsuits and skyrocketing malpractice premiums?

The malpractice system makes patients wait years to be compensated, does not compensate all patients who have been injured, and saddles many doctors with very high premiums.

7. Economic Revitalization

Does the proposal eliminate healthcare considerations from the purview of business, so businesses can focus on the core competencies? Will the new system guarantee total insurance portability? Will the proposal reduce labor-management conflict and permit hiring based on productivity and not fringe benefits?

Healthcare costs strain relationships between workers and their employers, and also create job-lock and wed-lock.

1. Guaranteed Coverage

Since 2000, the number of uninsured Americans has increased by 7 million. Today, 47 million Americans—including nearly 9 million children—are without health insurance. Almost two-thirds of the uninsured are full-time workers or live in households with at least one full-time worker. Most earn too little to afford insurance, yet of those uninsured nearly 28 percent—13 million Americans—earn over $60,000 a year. These people either opt not to get insurance or are prevented from getting it at a reasonable price because of preexisting medical conditions such as cancer. Even people who are quite well-to-do are falling through the cracks of our current system.

Consider Jason Levi, a 56-year-old Chicago-based financial adviser and stockbroker. Working out of his home, he invests millions of dollars on everything from the price of oil and other commodities to the price swings of stocks and bonds. Although he does very well for himself, Levi is not immune to health insurance problems. Several years ago, two basal-cell cancers were removed from Levi's wife's forearm. Such tumors are slow growing, rarely metastasize, and cause no symptoms unless they go untreated. Because basal cells grow on the surface of the skin, they are easily monitored and can be easily removed in an office procedure. Yet, because they are also labeled "cancers," Levi and his wife could not get health insurance. Luckily, Levi knows some wealthy, powerful people. One of his clients agreed to put Levi on his company's payroll, so that he and his wife would be in a group and qualify for the company's health insurance benefits.

Unlike Levi, Vicki Readling didn't have wealth or wealthy friends. In 2005, in a bold move, she decided to quit working for a North Carolina furniture manufacturer to become a real-estate agent. While she would make more money, about $60,000 per year, she forfeited her former employer's health plan and was left without any benefits. Through the Consolidated Omnibus Budget Reconciliation Act (COBRA), Readling temporarily extended her health insurance from her previous job as she searched for new individual coverage. A month into her search, Readling was diagnosed with breast cancer. As a result of her new cancer, many insurance companies would not cover her, and the ones that would had premiums over $27,000 per year and deductibles of $5,000. "I don't know which is worse, being told that I had cancer or finding that I could not get insurance," Vicki said. "What did I do wrong? I just don't understand how I could have fallen through this horrible, horrible crack."

While uninsured individuals often receive some healthcare, being uninsured usually means getting too little care when it's already too late. Lacking insurance, many people put off going to the doctor for fear of receiving a bill they can't pay. Some attempt to stretch out their medications to save money, even though taking pills every other day rather than twice a day can be deadly. A recent study found that when uninsured Americans are admitted to a hospital, they are 20 percent more likely to be admitted to the intensive care unit (ICU) with more serious conditions than insured patients, and, in the ICU, are 20 percent more likely to die. According to the Institute of Medicine,

18,000 Americans die prematurely each year because their lack of insurance prevents them from getting necessary healthcare interventions in time.

Aside from removing the moral stain of leaving 47 million Americans without health insurance, guaranteed coverage for all Americans would honor the economic contributions of the more than 20 million full-time workers who pay taxes but lack healthcare coverage because they can't afford it. With guaranteed coverage, rich and poor will all have a secure safety net: When we need healthcare, we will be able to get it.

Guaranteed coverage ensures that *all* Americans will receive a standard set of benefits without exception. It does not mean providing health insurance for 95 percent or 97 percent of the population. As Medicare and other countries' health systems have successfully demonstrated, 100 percent coverage is within our reach. Falling short of 100 percent is unacceptable.

The standard services guaranteed to Americans should be comparable to what their congressional representatives and senators receive. At a minimum, these benefits should include office and home visits, hospitalization, preventive screening tests, prescription drugs, some dental care, mental-health care, and physical and occupational therapies.

2. Effective Cost Controls

Guaranteeing coverage for all Americans is certainly the biggest and most important goal of a new healthcare system, but it is far from the only issue to be solved. There is also the sheer size of the bill. Healthcare costs are skyrocketing. In 1970, healthcare for an individual cost $356 per year. By 2006, it cost over $7,000. More than $1 out of every $6 spent in America goes to healthcare. Of the more than $2.7 trillion comprising the total federal budget, $1 out of $5 ($580 billion) goes to Medicare, Medicaid, and the State's Children's Health Insurance Program (SCHIP)—and that does not account for government spending on the National Institutes of Health (NIH), the Centers for Disease Control and Prevention (CDC), pandemic flu preparedness, the veterans' healthcare program, and a multitude of other health-related government services.

The cost of healthcare is hurting all of us. For state governments, the expenses associated with Medicaid and health insurance for state workers are overwhelming: They now account for nearly 32 percent of state budgets—and cost more than any other state expense. In 2000, Medicaid cost our nation $203 billion; by 2006 (the last year for which we have statistics), it had risen 60 percent to $321 billion. Over one-third of American states had Medicaid budget shortfalls in 2005. Consequently, in the last few years, forty-five states have cut those benefits not mandated by federal law. As healthcare costs have gone up, states have tightened Medicaid eligibility requirements. Between 2001 and 2004, when costs rose and the economy floundered, Tennessee responded by dropping 190,000 people from Medicaid and Texas cut 150,000 children from SCHIP. Meanwhile, states have also cut other public programs to pay for the costs of Medicaid. As a result, tuition at state colleges and universities has increased and cuts have been made in other programs for education, highways, the environment, and prisons.

Likewise, businesses and their workers feel the sting of rising healthcare costs. Between 2001 and 2005, health insurance premiums rose by 68 percent. In 2007, the average annual cost of employer-based health insurance for a family was over $12,000. In human terms, this means that the cost of providing one employee with family healthcare coverage is equivalent to the cost of hiring a second employee at minimum wage. This $12,000 figure constitutes roughly 25 percent of the median family income in the United States (about $49,000 in 2007). For too many of us, healthcare has simply become an economic impossibility.

Unable to afford this kind of overhead, businesses are responding by cutting the number of employees to whom they provide health insurance or reducing the comprehensiveness of that insurance. Between 2000 and 2006, the percentage of companies offering healthcare coverage to their employees fell from 69 percent to under 60 percent. Even with a growing population, the number of Americans covered by employer-based insurance declined by more than 5 million during these years, while the number of uninsured increased.

Meanwhile, families are paying ever more. The elderly pay nearly $1 out of every $4 of income for healthcare—*more* than they paid before Medicare. Between 1999 and 2005, workers' average contributions to their health insurance premiums increased 75 percent, while deductibles—the amount they pay before their insurance kicks in—increased 500 percent. A worker laid off when his company closed its last American factory and moved production to China articulated the problem clearly: "I have a mortgage, vehicle payments, heat, electricity. Right now I have a choice of taking [health] insurance or eating. So I chose eating." For many families, the choices are even harder.

Days before 5-year-old Kenny Main was diagnosed with acute leukemia, his father, a self-employed electrician in Florida, joined the National Association for the Self-Employed to purchase a health insurance policy for his family at $227 per month. The policy was inexpensive because it carried a $5,000 deductible. Kenny's treatment took eighteen months, and the bills eventually totaled over $500,000. The insurance company denied the Main's claims, paying only "a little bit here and a little bit there," while steadily increasing the premium. Between medical bills and insurance costs, the Mains were rapidly running out of money. When their premium checks bounced, the insurance company promptly cancelled their health insurance policy. Today the cost and structure of healthcare puts responsible but unlucky families in desperate straits.

It is important to distinguish between high healthcare *costs* and high healthcare *cost increases.* Through comprehensive reform, we can improve efficiency by decreasing excessive administrative expenses, eliminating waste, and reducing fraud. Such improvements can generate tens of billions of dollars each year in savings.

But the real worry is healthcare inflation. Every year for the past thirty years, healthcare costs have risen an average of 2.1 percent faster than the rate of economic growth. Each year an increasing amount of the GDP is going to healthcare. Today 16 percent of our GDP pays for healthcare, and by 2015 it will be just under 20 percent. If this trend continues, by 2028, over one-quarter of all the money in the American economy—to be precise, 28¢ of every $1—will be devoted to healthcare alone. Everything else we need and want, including housing, food, clothing, cars, fuel, entertainment, education, telephones, computers, vacations, movies, music, books, toys, flowers—you name it—will have to be squeezed out of the remaining 72¢.

In order to achieve guaranteed healthcare for all Americans, it is essential to reign in cost inflation. We have the power to change the slope of the curve so that healthcare does not consume an ever-rising share of the GDP. We can control the rate of healthcare cost inflation by developing cost-effective technologies, delivering care in the most cost-effective settings, and using the most cost-effective practices available.

While most of the financing for healthcare in the United States is provided to the general public through employer-based insurance, Medicaid, SCHIP, and Medicare are exceptions. But each of these is inefficient, inequitable, and, because of cost, increasingly unsustainable. Comprehensive reform must create a new financing vehicle that eliminates multiple financing mechanisms.

3. High-Quality, Coordinated Care

Even though Americans pay exorbitantly for healthcare coverage, the actual medical care we receive is nowhere close to the consistently high quality we expect and deserve. Study after study, and the experience of millions of Americans, tell us that far too many patients are victims of preventable medical errors and hospital-acquired infections. In many cases, patients are overtreated, undertreated, or treated with unproven drugs and technologies that increase costs without providing better health outcomes. In some cases, medical treatments exacerbate existing health problems or result in death.

In its 1999 report *To Err Is Human*, the Institute of Medicine estimated that as many as 98,000 Americans die each year from preventable medical errors. In 2006, Jasmine Gant, a 19-year-old from Fitchburg, Wisconsin, offered a human face to this statistic when she went into labor with her first child. Instead of getting the intravenous penicillin her physician ordered, she was mistakenly injected with an epidural anesthetic. Twenty minutes later she began to have seizures and could not be revived.

Unfortunately, such errors are far too common, even at America's best hospitals. Consider the story of Donald Berwick, who is one of the nation's leading experts on healthcare quality. A few years ago, Berwick's wife Ann, a competitive cross-country skier, had a sudden, unexplained loss of mobility. The Berwicks searched for a diagnosis and effective treatment at some of the best hospitals in America, including Harvard's Brigham and Women's Hospital and the Mayo Clinic. Despite having access to the best of American medicine, and even though Donald Berwick closely monitored his wife's treatment, Ann Berwick's saga was riddled with mistakes:

> One morning, a neurologist warned that Ann shouldn't get a certain kind of drug. By that afternoon, someone had given it to her. Another medication was discontinued by her doctor on her first day of admission [to the hospital], but the nurses continued to bring it every night for the next two weeks. Later, her doctors decided to put her through chemotherapy to try to stop the deterioration of her condition. "Time is of the essence," her doctor told her. The first dose [of chemotherapy] was given 60 hours later.

Don Berwick estimates that, in three months, his wife saw more than 100 doctors and was subject to numerous errors and near misses. The problem was not that she didn't have brilliant, dedicated doctors and nurses or the latest high-technology tests. The problem was the system—how the healthcare she received was organized and delivered.

Aside from having to deal with frightening medical errors, patients routinely acquire infections in hospitals, where new breeds of tenacious bugs resistant to almost all antibiotics can proliferate. According to the CDC, 5 percent of all patients admitted to hospitals acquire infections during their stay. At some of the larger hospitals in the United States the figure is as high as 10 percent. The result? Between 2 million and 3 million cases of life-threatening hospital-acquired infections and, according to the CDC, over 26,000 deaths per year. Almost all of these would have been preventable with the correct hand-washing and other procedures.

Hospital-acquired infections, late interventions, and medical errors are only the obvious problems affecting healthcare quality in the United States; the absence of optimal care is less evident. A recent study by the RAND think tank showed that Americans receive only 55 percent of recommended care. Patients don't necessarily receive even simple preventive treatments such as adult vaccines and cholesterol-lowering drugs. The federal government's Agency for Healthcare Research and Quality recently found that fewer than one out of three Americans with high blood pressure actually have the condition controlled adequately, even though high blood pressure can be easily monitored and effectively treated with inexpensive drugs.

Expensive treatments that are neither medically useful nor cost-effective drag down quality while driving up costs. Using an unproven expensive technology instead of a proven cheaper alternative increases costs without improving health or decreasing mortality. Brand-name drugs, which can cost five times as much as generic drugs that are equally effective, generate costs without medical benefits. A recent study of high-blood-pressure medications reported that none of the fancy new drugs—from angiotensin-converting enzyme inhibitors to angiotensin receptor blockers—were better than simple diuretics, and in some cases, they were worse. The traditional, low-dose diuretics prescribed for high blood pressure cost only pennies per pill because they have been off patent for decades. It is senseless to prescribe expensive drugs and treatments that are no better than less expensive, tried-and-true alternatives. But physicians do so far too often. Researchers at Stanford recently estimated that about 20 percent of the prescriptions physicians write are for drugs that have not been proven to have *any* therapeutic effect at all on the patient's condition. Another recent study showed that one-third of urologists were giving a very expensive drug to men with very early-stage prostate cancer despite the fact that the drug had never been shown to save lives or improve quality of life for patients with such early disease. Again, cost with no benefit.

Quality failures that drive up costs are also prevalent in medical procedures. The number of Caesarian sections performed on mothers varies widely: from 12.5 percent in Minneapolis to 25.6 percent in Miami and 26.4 percent in Fresno, California. This variation indicates that many C-sections are not medically necessary. Research shows that the greater use of C-sections for babies of normal birthweight has no benefits in terms of decreasing infant mortality or preserving the mother's health. Indeed, C-sections may actually cause slightly more problems, given the potential for infections and complications of the surgical wounds, but physicians perform them anyway, racking up costs twice as high as normal, vaginal, deliveries. Performing a C-section on a mother who intends to have another child also raises future costs: Each subsequent delivery by a woman who has undergone a C-section often requires the operation.

The list of high-cost, low-to-no-benefit treatments is long. In the 1990s, about 40,000 American women received bone marrow transplants for metastatic breast cancer, at a cost of about $100,000 each. These transplants, which were performed in the absence of any evidence of improved survival compared to regular chemotherapy, may have actually increased short-term deaths. And some intensive treatments for metastatic colon cancer cost $180,000 per patient but do not cure anyone, at best prolonging life an average of twenty to thirty weeks. Such cases of medical treatment without any proven benefits sap the nation's coffers, yet they continue to arise across the field.

A new American healthcare system must include quality controls that make delivery of healthcare consistently excellent. Myriad examples of excellent quality-control programs in other complex industries can serve as models. Virginia Mason Hospital in Seattle has adapted Toyota's lean production system to its standardized practices, resulting in a more efficient way of arranging medical instruments and permitting any employee to raise a concern about the quality of care. These quality-control programs succeed because they build accountability into their systems, something we frequently lack in American healthcare today.

Quality care ultimately requires the integration and coordination of care. Fragmented care is one of the greatest systemic flaws of health coverage today. We need the expertise of many physicians to ensure the best quality of care, but doctors tend to work separately in relative isolation. Consequently, patient care is adversely affected by poor communication, lack of coordination, and contradictory care plans. For instance, a typical breast cancer patient needs care from a surgeon, a radiation oncologist, and a medical oncologist, who provides chemotherapy. But the doctors frequently work separately, and the patient suffers as a result.

Consider the case of Joyce Wallis, a 47-year-old single woman working in Washington, D.C., far from her family and friends. She not only had to battle breast cancer but also faced problems and frustration caused by fragmented care. As she wrote:

> There is a confusion about my surgery. I have been asking if there will be any problems in the future if I get immediate reconstruction with an implant now and the possibility of my having to get radiation in the future on my axilla. And now they are telling me that implants and radiation do not work well together. And this is two days before the surgery! We may have to change my entire surgery and just do a single mastectomy without reconstruction, which means I would not have a breast for a very long time. I have not prepared for this at all. . . . I am upset that all of this was not communicated properly among all of the doctors and to me. I am mad and confused, but I am not quite sure what to do.

Clearly, a new American healthcare system must include a modernized delivery system. Fragmented care must be replaced by coordinated care that integrates physician services, hospital care, pharmacy services, vision care, home health services, and hospice care. We need a solid infrastructure to deliver effective care, incentives for efficiency and quality, and information systems that facilitate coordinated care.

To ensure an improved system of care, health insurers, physicians, and other healthcare providers must be accountable for keeping records, routinely reporting outcomes, and delivering high-quality, coordinated medical care. We know we need coordinated care, but as of now no one has determined the best way to integrate infrastructure, incentives, and information to deliver the highest quality efficiently. A successful system must ensure flexibility that stimulates innovation in the delivery of care, and providers need the freedom and incentives to try different approaches. The rise of HIV/AIDS in the 1980s and 1990s and the current obesity epidemic remind us that health problems as well as their treatments change. A successful American healthcare system must foster accountability and flexibility in order to effectively tackle healthcare problems as they arise.

4. Choice

Universal coverage, cost containment, and consistent quality are the three healthcare goals most widely acknowledged and championed. Even if it were possible to create a new American healthcare system that achieved these goals at the same cost as that of our current system, it is doubtful that most Americans would think of accepting it without being able to choose their physicians, hospitals, or insurance plans. Americans, especially those who suffer from serious or life-threatening diseases, consider wider choice and continuity to be essential elements of higher quality. Ultimately, choice must be a key goal of any healthcare system.

Choice does not merely encompass choices among insurance plans, physicians, and hospitals. The new American healthcare system must also give citizens the freedom to purchase extra healthcare benefits beyond the standard benefits that are guaranteed to all. We are used to being able to spend our money on what we want. If we want a fancier car, a smaller, faster computer with more memory, or a luxury vacation, we can pay the extra cost for such things and skimp somewhere else if necessary. The key is that it is our decision. And so it should be with healthcare. If people want brand-name drugs, a wider choice of eyeglasses, more mental-health benefits, or access to alternative medicine, they should be able to buy it. Some may want to pay for house calls or unlimited email access to a doctor. Probably the most important option for a patient is the ability to get a second opinion and then to choose the best doctor for any serious illness. Americans certainly deserve the freedom to buy additional healthcare benefits, as long as everyone has high-quality standard coverage.

Today, however, choice is limited even for insured Americans. Even with employer-provided insurance, fewer than half of workers are able to choose their health insurance plan and doctor. Meanwhile (because the reimbursements paid are so low), physicians frequently turn away Medicaid patients, and even Medicare patients are beginning to find themselves with fewer options. An effective healthcare system should make these limitations obsolete.

5. Fair Funding

Fairness in paying for a new American healthcare system is essential. Lower-income Americans should not bear the burden of subsidizing the rich. Instead, each of us should assume responsibility for paying our fair share. Those who can afford to pay more for healthcare should provide the social safety net for poor or retired individuals, children, and sick and disabled people.

6. Reasonable Dispute Resolution

Disputes over incidents of alleged medical malpractice hurt both patients and physicians alike. Patients must wait years to resolve claims, and doctors pay increasingly outrageous amounts of money for malpractice insurance. Numerous studies have shown that the majority of patients who suffer a medical error are not compensated, while a select few win outsized awards. On average, patients must wait nearly five years to receive payment from a malpractice case, with cases related to the delivery of a baby taking an average of six years.

Often, the cost of physicians' malpractice premiums goes up regardless of the quality of care they deliver to patients. Premiums rise whether or not patients sue their doctors or the doctors harm their patients. Between 2000 and 2004, medical malpractice premiums increased an average of 120 percent; in 2004, obstetricians in Dade County, Florida, paid an average of $277,000 in malpractice premiums, while some neurosurgeons in New

York paid over $300,000. Yet during the same period, malpractice insurance companies paid out only 10 percent more. According to experts, malpractice premiums have more to do with the financial practices and priorities of insurance companies than with the frequency or cost of medical errors.

Incremental attempts to solve the problem, such as putting caps on pain-and-suffering awards, have not been effective: They do not compensate injured patients more quickly or fairly, and they do not succeed in holding down doctors' premiums. We need to find a better way to resolve malpractice claims when we undertake comprehensive reform of our healthcare system. Compensating patients who have been tragically injured must cease to be a lottery system of compensation, and the few bad physicians who repeatedly harm patients must be prohibited from practicing. But for the rest, there should be a focus on ensuring that the system protects patients from needless harm rather than on compensating them after a mistake has happened. This approach would not only reduce defensive medicine but also revive physicians' attitudes toward practicing.

7. Economic Revitalization

The 800-pound gorilla in the room is the impact of healthcare costs on the economy. The biggest impact is on average working people. Except for the Hollywood writers' strike in 2008, almost all of the strikes and labor/management conflicts in the United States over the past decade have been related to healthcare. Demands for healthcare benefits have been at the top of the agenda in strikes staged by grocery workers in southern California; teachers in suburban Chicago; nurses at the Robert Wood Johnson University Hospital in New Jersey; mechanics at the helicopter manufacturer Sikorsky; janitors in Houston, Texas; and the United Auto Workers during their recent negotiations with the car companies. Given the state of national healthcare, so-called fringe benefits can no longer be considered "fringe." According to the Bureau of Labor Statistics, 30 percent of America's total worker compensation now goes to benefits rather than to take-home pay.

Healthcare costs are also a major distorting factor in hiring decisions. Lucy Snowe, for example, worked as a lecturer at an Ivy League university for years and was given a series of annual contracts rather than being hired as a full-time, tenure-track professor solely because healthcare and other benefits would have made her compensation package cost the university a third more.

Such an example is far from exceptional. To reduce their labor costs, companies avoid hiring older workers, who typically need more healthcare and drive up the insurance premiums. Similarly, many organizations hire part-time employees to avoid paying benefits. The firm that had provided security guards to Chicago's O'Hare International Airport for more than a decade was significantly underbid recently by a company that did not offer their guards healthcare benefits. For other employers, high healthcare costs enhance the allure of outsourcing.

There is also "job-lock," as noted in Chapter 1. Aside from the literal cost and availability of healthcare, many people are so afraid of losing their health coverage that they remain locked in jobs or make job choices based on whether or not healthcare insurance is offered. Vicki Readling is a case in point: Underwriting makes it very hard for individuals like her to afford premiums. Indeed, some employees stay in jobs that provide health coverage even when they qualify for higher-paying jobs without coverage or when they want to start businesses of their own. Job-lock affects people high and low—even well-educated, well-paid executives. If, like Jason Levi, an executive's spouse has a chronic illness or her child has survived cancer, she might be disqualified from health insurance at a new company. Ultimately, job-lock stifles American innovation and entrepreneurism, two long-standing features of our national identity.

Finally, there is what might be called "wed-lock." Some people stay in dysfunctional or unhappy marriages to retain their spouse's health coverage. Conversely, individuals like Vicki Readling may hesitate to marry for fear of saddling their new partner with a host of insurance issues and possibly debt. As Vicki confessed, "I am scared to get married because I don't have insurance. If I have to go to the hospital and I can't pay my hospital bills, what happens? Do they go after him?"

Unshackling business from the burden of providing healthcare benefits is a necessary goal for a new American healthcare system. Comprehensive reform must sever the link between employment and health insurance so that healthcare obligations no longer determine hiring decisions and business priorities. We need to implement comprehensive healthcare reform that revitalizes American business, rather than maintaining a system that stifles innovation.

SETTING CONCRETE GOALS for a new American healthcare system is vitally important, but it is perhaps even more important that citizens find the courage to demand *comprehensive* reform of the system. Our system is so fundamentally and irreparably flawed that *incremental* healthcare reforms can only exacerbate the chaotic and exorbitantly expensive services we receive today. We need to solve all of these problems, not make vain attempts to patch up a few.

By definition, incremental reform does not even endeavor to solve all of the problems besetting our healthcare system. Indeed, quick fixes such as covering all children or instituting electronic medical records cannot solve even one problem *completely*. The issue here is not that drug and insurance companies, hospitals, physicians, lawyers, and government officials are all evil, or that a single part of the system is a bit out of joint or in need of straightening. On the contrary, even if all the players were honest and reasonable, and we could shore up some of the shaky foundation, American healthcare would still be a mess. It is the structure that is dysfunctional—not the individuals or organizations involved. Everything is out of whack, from the motivations behind insurance companies' actions, to the ways in which hospitals and physicians organize the delivery of care, to individual patients, to the inadequate ways in which new medical interventions are evaluated.

Ensuring coverage for the 47 million uninsured Americans won't solve most of our healthcare problems. Coverage alone cannot make the system sustainable: We have to *simultaneously* address other critical issues, such as the cost and quality of care, to create and maintain a system that will continue to serve all Americans well into the future.

Some people, especially experts who have lots of experience in healthcare, have a negative gut reaction to the idea of comprehensive reform. From their perspective, completely restructuring America's entire healthcare system is too much to ask. But Americans are not so jaded or pessimistic. We have made major changes in the past, and we are willing to do the same again. In the last century, three comprehensive changes of profound significance were brought about on American soil: Civil rights became law, women got the right to vote, and Social Security was enacted. In each case, change began with a vision and with definitive goals in mind. Before discussing *whether* comprehensive reform can happen, it is necessary to decide *what* reform is needed.

A sustainable American healthcare system is within our reach, but it's up to us to transform the goals of the proposed plan into reality. To incite successful reform, we need to clearly comprehend the key causes of our healthcare crisis. Decisive goals for the future and a clear understanding of the present will prepare citizens for engaging in the political process and force our representatives to do something brave and innovative, rather than muddling along with a failing system.

CHAPTER 3

History and Havoc: Diagnosis of the Problem

One way to grasp the scope of the American healthcare calamity is through comparisons with other rich countries of the world. In the United States, 16 percent of the annual GDP is spent on healthcare—*substantially more* than any other prosperous country. By comparison, Germany spends 10.9 percent of its GDP on healthcare, France spends 10.5 percent, Norway 9.7 percent, Sweden 9.1 percent, Denmark 8.9 percent, Israel 8.4 percent, and Britain 8.3 percent. Because the United States has a larger GDP per person, spending a higher percentage of our GDP reflects more dollars spent per person. Yet our healthcare system does not stack up, and we have poorer health outcomes to show for all of our exorbitant spending. We spend more on healthcare but get less of life.

Why is the American healthcare system so riddled with coverage problems, high costs, inconsistent quality, malpractice suits, and the rest? How can we fail to provide healthcare insurance for 16 percent of our population, deliver uneven quality to the 84 percent of Americans who are insured, and yet pay 50 percent more per person than countries like France, Israel, and Britain, which cover all of their citizens? Why does the United States rate more poorly than its European counterparts in coverage, cost, and quality of healthcare?

Are we less efficient? Are our physicians cavalier about quality? Are they less knowledgeable or greedier than European physicians? Do they work fewer hours? Are they forced to work with older equipment—older MRI scanners, older heart monitors, and older computers—that detracts from their productivity?

Or is our healthcare system a mess because of the hard-hearted managed-care companies? If we didn't have so many unscrupulous malpractice lawyers, would we be in such a bind? Can we chalk up most of our problems to the greedy pharmaceutical industry and blood-sucking insurance companies?

None of these explanations pass the sniff test. None of them reveal the underlying factors responsible for our healthcare crisis. Nor can we blame an overdeveloped tolerance for inefficiency, waste, poor quality, and government bureaucracies. And the problems we experience with coverage, cost, and quality certainly cannot be blamed on a lack of cutting-edge technology.

The underlying problem is the *structure* of the American healthcare system. Given a blank sheet of paper, no one would ever design our current system. And no one *did* design it. It grew out of a series of accidents that have left us with a chaotic, unstable, and unsustainable healthcare system. The fact that most Americans get health coverage through their employer is the consequence of historical exigencies rather than careful consideration of efficiency, equity, and sustainability. The fragmented delivery system, driven by thousands of small physician practices, is a remnant of the horse-and-buggy era, ill-suited to the twenty-first century.

The crumbling of the two supporting pillars of the system—the *financing* that pays for healthcare and the *delivery* that actually provides services to patients—threatens the whole healthcare system. Their deterioration explains our problems with access, cost, quality, and malpractice. As decades of psychological research indicate, placing well-intentioned, hard-working people into a terribly dysfunctional structure will create a mess. This is the story of America's healthcare system.

Problems with Financing Healthcare

Employer-Based Insurance

Despite seeming well entrenched, employer-based health coverage is a fairly recent phenomenon. It started in the United States in the late 1800s when mining, lumber, and railroad companies began to provide healthcare for their workers. Luring physicians to remote places, companies guaranteed to pay them for treating sick and injured employees, so that employees could return to work.

The big boost in employment-based insurance came during World War II because of workers who could not receive pay raises despite pouring sweat into war production. To placate workers and to give employers a means with which to attract labor, the War Labor Board permitted companies to offer fringe benefits worth up to 5 percent of wages. Soon after, the federal government exempted health insurance benefits from personal and business taxation. For workers, a dollar in health insurance benefits was suddenly more valuable than a dollar pay increase, a subsidy that became even more desirable as wages rose and worker income tax brackets rose with them. Meanwhile, health insurance expenses became tax deductible for businesses.

Right after World War II, state Blue Cross and Blue Shield organizations controlled about 75 percent of all private healthcare insurance. As nonprofit organizations, they set premiums through community rating, charging all companies and workers the same premiums, regardless of age or other risk factors, such as whether a person smoked. With the community rating of many companies, cross-subsidization resulted: Workers at one company subsidized those at another, the young supplemented the old, the healthy supplemented the sick, and executives subsidized lower-wage workers. Consequently, employment-based insurance in the early days created quasi-social insurance.

In those early days, employment-based insurance was able to provide broad-based health security to such a large number of workers, managers, and executives because they were all part of *one* insurance pool. Efficient and low-cost health insurance depends upon *pooling* a large number of healthy and unhealthy people to purchase coverage. Pooling large numbers of people makes costs predictable for insurance companies. Because so many people contribute payments to the system, the insurer is made more resilient: An insurance company can continue to thrive even when some of the people in the pool need expensive medical services. Large pools also divide the cost of administrative fees—underwriting, marketing, and sales—among a larger number of people, thereby making these costs a smaller fraction of the premium. Within a large pool, moreover, it is easier and more economical to develop expertise or hire consultants to advise on how to efficiently shape the insurance policies so as to lower costs.

For a long time, employment-based insurance seemed a success. Between 1940 and 1950, the number of Americans with private health insurance increased seven-fold from about 20 million to over 140 million. By the late 1970s, employment-based health insurance had reached its apex, with 85 percent of civilian, noninstitutionalized Americans covered by some form of private healthcare insurance.

But even at its best, employment-based health insurance was defective. After World War II, for-profit, commercial insurers started aggressively entering healthcare. By offering risk-rating premiums, for-profit insurers started enticing companies away from Blue Cross and Blue Shield; they gave lower rates to employers with younger, healthier workers. And so began a vicious, self-reinforcing cycle. Because the pool of companies was now smaller, with fewer healthy workers, risk increased along with underwriting, marketing, and sales costs per enrollee. And as healthcare premiums increased, companies had an even greater incentive to exit the larger Blue Cross/Blue Shield pool. Additional policies, such as the Employee Retirement Income Security Act (ERISA) of 1974, which removed even more workers from the large insurance pool, further eroded the system's integrity.

Today, employment-based insurance as social insurance has essentially vanished. Left behind is a terribly inefficient system that undermines widespread coverage and costs far too much. Because each place of employment has to purchase health insurance on its own, administrative costs are exorbitant—estimated to exceed $120 billion per year, without counting the money that employers spend to manage healthcare benefits for their employees. Alain Enthoven and Victor Fuchs, two prominent American health economists, vividly describe the magnitude of the financial impact of employer healthcare:

> The need for more than 850 insurance companies to see and contract with millions of employers, underwriting each one, adds greatly to administrative overhead costs. Typically, administrative costs are on the order of 11 percent of premium, and this does not include the costs to employers to purchase and manage healthcare spending, including armies of consultants, benefits managers, and brokers. To understand how this could be different, consider that Kaiser Permanente signs one annual contract for the coverage of more than 400,000 employees and dependents with the California Public Employees Retirement System (CalPERS) and CalPERS' administrative costs are on the order of 0.5 percent of premium.

That extra 10.5 percent of premium from administration—the difference between 11 percent of premium for typical plans and

0.5 percent for a single big employer—increases costs without providing real health benefits.

Aside from its inefficiency, the employer-based health insurance system has become grossly unfair. Higher costs fall disproportionately onto small and low-wage businesses. With small risk pools, fewer employees to absorb the administrative costs, and the inability to hire consultants to negotiate better deals, premiums for employees of small employers have become prohibitively high. Consequently, only 45 percent of small companies (those with three to twenty-four workers) provide health insurance, while 68 percent of large firms (1,000 to 4,999 employees) do so. As these administrative costs hike health insurance premiums, offering health insurance becomes increasingly difficult for employers with lower average wages. For a company paying workers $10 per hour, providing family health insurance costs more than half the hourly wage. Individual coverage alone results in 20 percent of hourly wage. In the low-wage retail sector only 43 percent of companies provide health coverage, compared to 76 percent of higher-wage manufacturers.

As health insurance costs rise, hiring and firing decisions are increasingly driven by healthcare costs rather than by productivity considerations, and more and more employees face job-lock.

Employer-provided healthcare coverage is unsustainable. Between 2001 and 2006, the number of American workers increased by nearly 8 million, yet the number of Americans with employer-based coverage stayed the same.

Increasing costs and decreasing coverage aren't the only factors bringing the employer-based healthcare system to its knees. The federal government has also taken a huge hit because of this financing mechanism, which not only doesn't require employees to pay income taxes on the healthcare benefits they receive but also allows employers to deduct them from their taxes as expenses. The U.S. Treasury loses in excess of $200 billion per year because of this tax break—almost double the mortgage deduction.

Aside from diverting needed funds from the government, the structure of the tax deduction creates significant social inequities. A very regressive tax break, the deduction helps rich, high-income employees far more than lower-income workers, even in terms of employer coverage. The Lewin consulting group has estimated that for workers earning less than $30,000 annually, the tax break on health insurance is worth $725, but for those earning $100,000 or more, the very same insurance policy is worth almost four times as much in tax relief: $2,800. It is no longer an option to maintain so skewed a system of financing healthcare. Something's got to give.

Medicaid and SCHIP

In the late 1950s, as employer-based insurance was expanding, it became obvious that even if it worked perfectly, many people—the unemployed, older retirees, disabled Americans—would be left out. After nearly a decade of national discussion and debate, on July 30, 1965, President Johnson signed the legislation creating Medicaid and Medicare. Over thirty years later, the Balanced Budget Act of 1997 established SCHIP, a program that provides coverage to millions of uninsured children.

Medicaid and SCHIP are programs shared between the federal and state governments that provide coverage for Americans who cannot afford to pay for healthcare: the poor, the unemployed, the disabled, and children. (Medicaid also pays for much of the nursing-home care for the elderly.) Most of the funding for Medicaid and SCHIP comes from the federal government, which also sets core benefits and eligibility requirements. States can provide additional benefits, expand eligibility requirements, and administer the programs. Medicaid currently covers 38 million Americans, and SCHIP covers 6 million children to the tune of more than $300 billion per year. However, like employer-based insurance, Medicaid and SCHIP are inefficient, inequitable, and increasingly unsustainable.

Medicaid and SCHIP inefficiencies arise both from administrative costs for determining eligibility and from substantial fraud on the part of healthcare providers. The application process for Medicaid is daunting. In New York State, Medicaid applicants are advised by the agency's website to bring the following information to an interview:

- Proof of age, such as a birth certificate
- Proof of citizenship or alien status
- Recent paycheck stubs (if the individual is working)
- Proof of income from sources such as Social Security, Supplemental Security Income (SSI), Veterans Administration (VA) benefits, and retirement benefits
- Any bank books and insurance policies in the individual's possession

- Proof of residence, such as a rent receipt or landlord statement
- An insurance benefit card or the policy (if the individual has any other health insurance)
- A Medicare benefit card

It costs as much for state employees to review, verify, and approve the enrollment of a single child in Medicaid or SCHIP as it does to pay for two months of healthcare premiums. The process for reviewing adults is even more expensive because they are subject to more restrictions. And further compounding the initial enrollment costs is the constant churning of people going on and off Medicaid again and again, as well as changes in administrative procedures that require additional reviews. In New York, for instance, the average time on Medicaid is just over nine months.

Extensive eligibility requirements keep many needy people off government-subsidized health programs. Researchers at the Urban Institute estimate that a total of 11 million uninsured Americans are eligible for Medicaid or SCHIP, but are not enrolled. Nearly 6 million of them are children. The administrative costs just for determining eligibility—not including payments for the actual delivery of healthcare services, auditing, and other administrative tasks—could cover one extra person for every six Medicaid beneficiaries. This is cost without benefit.

Ironically, while states spend substantial sums to screen applicants for Medicaid, they spend far less on oversight of physicians, hospitals, and other healthcare providers. James Mehmet, the retired chief investigator of Medicaid fraud in New York State, recently reported that 10 percent of the state's Medicaid dollars were spent on outright fraudulent claims, while 20 percent to 30 percent more were siphoned off by unnecessary spending that is not necessarily criminal. In 2004, state investigators visited just 95 of the 140,000 different Medicaid providers in New York State.

The costs associated with fraud and enrollment point to fundamental flaws in Medicaid and SCHIP, but the relentless increases in healthcare costs across the board pose an even bigger problem. Medicaid now constitutes the single largest part of state budgets, and its continuous expansion threatens other worthy programs. Between 2000 and 2006, the cost of Medicaid rose nearly 60 percent, while state revenues rose less than 25 percent. In 2007, the National Governors Association reported that all healthcare accounted for 32 percent of state budgets—the single largest portion of total state spending. When Medicaid costs increase above general inflation and above tax receipts, money has to come from somewhere to make up the difference. (Most states cannot go into deficit.) So other services are cut from the budget. State transportation programs, funding for jails, and environmental programs have all been targeted, but since 2000 higher education has taken the biggest hit. In 2004 alone, states raised tuition and fees at their colleges and universities by an average of 14 percent. This creates a *healthcare cost–education trade-off:* Increased Medicaid costs squeeze families trying to send their children to colleges and universities and impede job retraining for adults returning to school.

This trade-off between healthcare costs and education is not an isolated occurrence. The National Governors Association has cautioned that Medicaid cost increases projected through 2017 will significantly strain state budgets and force cuts in other programs. And that warning came *before* the recent economic downturn.

The costs of Medicaid and SCHIP unduly burden state budgets, but even apart from that, they are inequitable. Although most of the money for Medicaid and SCHIP comes from the federal government, the benefits and requirements for coverage for Medicaid and SCHIP vary from state to state. In five states, children whose parents earn 250 percent of the federal poverty level or more (about $50,000 per year for a family of four) can be enrolled in these programs, while in other states only those children whose parents earn less than 133 percent of the poverty level (about $26,700) are eligible—even though SCHIP is supposed to cover children up to 200 percent of the poverty level. Moreover, in some states, adults with incomes at 200 percent of the federal poverty level are eligible for Medicaid, while in thirty-five states family income must be below the poverty line for eligibility. In fourteen states, parents with incomes at half the poverty level are ineligible for these federal programs.

Of the millions of Americans ineligible for Medicaid assistance, 70 percent are full-time workers or members of households in which at least one adult is a full-time worker. An additional 11 percent of the uninsured work part time or are dependents of these workers. These Americans are trapped. Their wages are so low that their employers cannot practically provide coverage, or, like Vicki Readling, they are self-employed and health insurance premiums are prohibitive. Yet these citizens dutifully contribute taxes that support Medicaid and SCHIP. We need a new American healthcare system that buoys up all of our citizens, one that encourages and rewards hard work.

Medicare

Medicare offers guaranteed coverage for the elderly, the disabled, and people with chronic renal disease. Enormously popular, it boasts more satisfied customers than any other health program in America. Since its inception, Medicare has added coverage for important services, including preventive care and prescription drugs. Well hidden from its beneficiaries, however, are defects that threaten to destroy the program.

Many people praise Medicare for its efficiency. It devotes only 3–4 percent of its expenditures to administration, so it certainly seems more efficient than most private insurance companies. And it's true that Medicare has fewer costs associated with underwriting, marketing, and sales. However, the figures do not tell the whole story. Medicare is challenged by one of the major problems facing Medicaid: Its low administrative costs permit fraud and fail to address other important issues associated with efficiency.

The 10 percent fraud level in Medicaid exists in Medicare, for the same reason. Both programs need to do more than process bills. A successful healthcare financing mechanism must invest in oversight and auditing to ensure that hospitals properly bill patients, that physicians provide the services they bill for, and that home healthcare agencies actually deliver services to patients. Oversight and auditing constitutes administrative costs. In 1996, the last year there was a report on Medicare fraud, the Inspector General of the Department of Health and Human Services estimated that Medicare made about $23.2 billion worth of improper payments (over 10 percent of total Medicare costs) due to insufficient or absent documentation, incorrect billing, and billing for excluded services. Clearly something is missing from the equation. Merrill Matthews of the Council for Affordable Health Insurance best summarized the situation when he noted:

> While everyone wants health insurance administrative costs to be as low as possible, that should mean as low as possible while still adequately adjudicating claims to ensure that insurers are paying only what they should. Medicare doesn't do that. As a result, Medicare is paying claims it shouldn't—and, ironically, making its administrative cost ratio look more favorable!

Maintaining excessively low administrative costs also means that big problems simply do not get addressed. For many years, Medicare's data on so-called indirect practice costs, which account for as much as 50 percent of office costs, have been "outdated." Medicare payments to medical practices don't reflect factors that have driven these costs down. Information technology has replaced administrative assistants, and office procedures have supplanted the need to send samples to laboratories. Updating Medicare's figures would require spending $3 million every few years to survey physicians' practices for their spending patterns. In the grand scheme of things, the cost to do so is minuscule, less than 0.001 percent of the Medicare budget. But Medicare, despite the potential of such an investment to reduce costs and pay physicians more accurately, refuses to do so. Why? According to the experts, its refusal stems from an effort to keep administrative costs down.

Even more harmful to Medicare is the huge variation in payments for particular medical services across the country. Payments for the same services are lower in Tennessee and Utah than in New York and Florida. While payments must vary based on location (after all, rent for office space in New York City is substantially higher than rent in Salt Lake City), Medicare's variations extend far beyond differences in the cost of living. An uncomplicated coronary artery bypass graft, or CABG, costs over $21,000 at the Mayo Clinic in Minnesota but is nearly 50 percent more expensive at Massachusetts General Hospital in Boston. Massachusetts General Hospital is a fantastic institution, but it seems doubtful that given a choice—and responsibility for the bill—most rational people would pay $9,000 more to get a heart operation there than at the Mayo Clinic. Yet changing such geographic imbalances in Medicare payments has proven impossible. Every time an attempt is made to address these imbalances, powerful members of Congress from high-cost states argue for their constituents, and the idea gets shelved.

By law, Medicare covers medical treatments that are "reasonable and necessary," but no formal definition of this phrase exists. In lieu of exact guidance, Medicare traditionally pays for drugs and devices approved by the Food and Drug Administration (FDA). But FDA approvals are based on whether or not a drug or device is "safe and effective," which, in turn, is usually determined by a drug's ability to better treat a condition than a placebo in a clinical trial. For the FDA, "effectiveness" does not mean that a drug is better than other drugs that do the same thing, or that the improvement in one drug over another is worth the cost. Rather, it simply means that a particular drug is better than nothing. Medicare thus ends up paying for a lot of expensive medicine without determining whether the added costs actually improve the quality or length of life.

Consider Erbitux, a drug used to treat metastatic colon cancer for roughly $40,000. Incapable of curing patients, on average it extends life just seven weeks. Avastin, another colon cancer drug capable of prolonging life for two to five months, but not of providing anyone a cure, costs about $50,000 per patient. Medicare covers the cost of both of these treatments.

The combination of continued payments for unproven tests and treatments, fraud, and uncorrected payment problems—along with the baby boom—threatens to bankrupt our country. In 1966, its first year of operation, Medicare covered 19 million Americans at a cost of $3.3 billion—less than 0.4 percent of our GDP. In 2006, by contrast, Medicare provided healthcare coverage for about 43 million Americans at a cost of just over $400 billion—fully 3.1 percent of the GDP. By 2030, 20 percent of the

U.S. population, 79 million Americans, will receive Medicare and consume 6.5 percent of our GDP: That's $1 of every $15 spent.

According to the Congressional Budget Office, Medicare and Medicaid account for 22.9 percent of all federal spending today. By 2017 these programs will consume nearly 33 percent of all federal spending. Unless we make some dramatic changes, by 2050 Medicare and Medicaid will consume more than *all* federal taxes. By 2080 Medicare *alone* will consume all federal taxes. At this rate, there will be no money available for any other government functions—defense, highways, scientific research, national parks, education, the environment, or the arts. Ironically, these projections are based on what health policy experts acknowledge to be unrealistically conservative estimates—estimates, that is, on a rate of increased government health spending that is significantly below what has occurred in the last three decades.

Making Medicare financially stable over the next seventy-five years would require doubling taxes or cutting benefits in half *today*. No wonder an editorial in the *New York Times* quipped that "[e]ven in fantasy, no one has yet come up with a way to pay for Medicare."

Problems with Healthcare Delivery

The problems of financing our healthcare system through Medicare, Medicaid, SCHIP, and employer-based healthcare insurance tell only half of the story. We have not only a broken financing system for healthcare but a broken delivery system.

The American healthcare delivery system is an antiquated cottage industry. Healthcare is still delivered the way medicine was delivered in the nineteenth century. Indeed, few people think of it as a *system*, to the extent that the word connotes any sense of organization and coherent structure. Instead, healthcare in this country is delivered through tens of thousands of small, independent, uncoordinated physician practices that are largely paid piece-rate to care for people whose major health problems are heart disease, cancer, diabetes, and other chronic conditions. This highly fragmented, uncoordinated arrangement might have been effective when doctors dealt primarily with acute problems, but today, when chronic illness is the biggest problem, such fragmentation leads to poor healthcare outcomes. When patients see multiple doctors who keep different medical records and require them to visit multiple facilities, it is nearly impossible for them to receive efficient, affordable quality care.

Efficient delivery of high-quality healthcare requires the three *I*'s: infrastructure, incentives, and information. We need an infrastructure that facilitates the integration of services and collaboration among numerous healthcare providers. We need a new incentive system that discourages quantity as a measure of quality. And we need a way to make healthcare decisions based on information about the effectiveness of tests and treatments, because the current system fails to produce critical information and deliver it to healthcare providers. Furthermore, infrastructure, incentives, and information must be synchronized. Outmoded incentives exacerbate fragmented delivery of care;

fragmented infrastructure undermines development and dissemination of the right information.

Coordination and Integration of Care

In 1900, medical care was provided by independent family physicians. People came to their doctors with broken bones, fevers, infections, and other acute problems. Ordinary patients did not have multiple health problems that required armfuls of medication—and, in any case, there were few effective interventions available for such problems.

Today, this approach to medicine is not just antiquated, it is harmful. Healthcare now centers on chronic illness. Thanks to the tremendous advances of modern medicine, patients are capable of surviving heart attacks, cancer, emphysema, and diabetes. Accordingly, they live on to contract new illnesses. Currently, over 133 million Americans live with chronic health conditions. Among Americans 65 years and older, 75 percent have two or more chronic conditions, and 20 percent have five or more. Obesity creates and exacerbates a constellation of health problems, from high blood pressure and heart disease to diabetes. When people with a chronic illness, such as heart disease, contract another medical problem, such as cancer or a serious infection, care becomes more complex and requires coordination among many different physicians and other caregivers. At present, 70 percent of all health expenditures are for the treatment of chronic conditions.

Scientific advances have complicated the practice of medicine. After World War II, there were only eight antibiotics and no antiviral agents available. Today, there are over one-hundred-twenty antibiotics and more than twenty antiviral agents. After World War II, we could treat cancer with radiation or four chemotherapy agents. Today, sixty-eight different anticancer agents are available, not to mention the anti-nausea medications and other treatments prescribed for the side effects of chemotherapy. Only decades ago, we had no drugs to treat high cholesterol. Today, there are seven different classes of drugs on the market capable of lowering cholesterol.

With ever more choices, physicians need to know a great deal more. But it is virtually impossible for an individual physician to keep up with the literature in even one area of medicine, let alone all of medicine's advances. On average, each month 4,000 English-language articles are published about cancer, with 500 or so on breast cancer alone. This proliferation of information motivates more and more physicians to become specialists. Four out of every five American physicians are specialists today. Within each specialty there are numerous subspecialties. Physicians are no longer just internists but cardiologists, some of whom specialize even further, performing only catheterizations or cardiac echoes, while others deal only with rhythm disorders.

As a result of increased specialization, most patients have multiple physicians. The typical Medicare patient sees seven different physicians each year, five of whom are specialists. Medicare patients with chronic conditions see even more doctors: eleven physicians working in seven different practices. Patients with five or more chronic conditions see approximately fourteen different physicians a year.

In the past, hospitals facilitated the coordination of care. In the 1960s, patients who suffered a heart attack frequently stayed in the hospital for twenty-one days or more. The cardiologist, lung specialist, and diabetes expert, as well as a patient's primary care physician, would come to the hospital to make rounds in the morning. Over a period of weeks, they would all have a chance to talk about how to manage the patient's care, and a single patient chart was shared among them. Today, by contrast, a patient will spend only a few days in the hospital, a "hospitalist" rather than the primary care physician is likely to manage the patient's hospital care, and there are few opportunities for the multiple physicians to discuss the patient together. With shorter hospital stays, most healthcare is delivered in a doctor's office or in specialized facilities outside of hospitals, such as centers for dialysis, physical therapy, and surgery. In such dispersed settings, it is difficult to coordinate care among physicians. Given the lack of shared electronic medical records, the potential for disasters due to duplication of treatments, conflicting orders, and medical errors is much higher.

Consider a patient who develops breast cancer. The journey might begin when her primary care physician feels a lump or orders a routine mammogram. She then sees a radiologist for the mammogram and maybe undergoes a biopsy at the radiology center. A pathologist at a different facility reads the biopsy slides. A surgeon removes the lump from her breast, after which a medical oncologist administers chemotherapy, and a radiation oncologist gives radiation therapy at the hospital. By the end of her treatment, the patient has seen six physicians at several offices and centers. For each visit, the patient is typically responsible for bringing all of her information, including her surgical and pathology reports, X-rays, CT scans, lab tests, and medical history.

Physicians rarely work together. In 2004, Americans visited physicians more than 1 billion times. A third of these visits were made to physicians who practice alone—solo practitioners—and another third were made to physicians in small groups of two to four physicians. Half of all physician visits are to physicians other than a patient's primary care physician. Surprisingly, the majority of these visits are self-referrals by patients, meaning that they are not coordinated among physicians. And only about 20 percent of physicians have electronic medical records to facilitate coordination of patient care. The coordination of this care between physicians and the increasingly important groups of nonphysician healthcare providers such as visiting nurses, pharmacists, respiratory and physical therapists, podiatrists, and hospice caregivers is similarly messy. When the American Society of Clinical Oncologists recently assessed the quality of cancer care, breast cancer patients listed referral and coordination of care as the worst category of care, and colon cancer patients reported it as second worst. Among breast cancer patients, coordination of care was marked as good quality only a paltry 13 percent of the time.

High-quality care requires an infrastructure that ensures coordination of care: Patients need to get proven tests and treatments in the most appropriate setting, whether that means going to a hospital, a physician's office, or a specialized center or staying at home for healthcare. Healthcare providers must work as a team to provide coordinated care, sharing the same care plan and medical record for a patient. Coordinated care also requires periodic reviews of costs and benefits to see how they can be improved. In addition, physicians and other caregivers must learn about updated and new treatments. Today, we are saddled with a system from the nineteenth century: a series of physicians who work alone, providing care, ordering tests, and delivering treatments as each one sees fit.

Payment for Care

When the fragmented healthcare system we have today started to take shape in the late nineteenth century, physicians had individual practices, and patients paid fees to their doctors directly. Despite the enormous growth in the size and complexity of American healthcare over the last century, fee-for-service remains the dominant model of payment. About 80 percent of Medicare patients participate in the traditional fee-for-service program. Of those people who have employment-based insurance, 60 percent are enrolled in preferred provider organizations, or PPOs. Physicians who work for these PPOs typically agree to accept a set fee as payment for particular services, so they are often referred to as in-network, "preferred" physicians. (Most other employer-provided health insurance policies also pay doctors set fees.)

Setting certain fees for particular services encourages physicians and hospitals to work efficiently, in a narrow sense, because they increase their profit by delivering a specific service cheaply. However, the fee-for-service model also encourages doctors to see more patients in the office, to perform more surgical operations, colonoscopies, lung function tests, and other procedures, and to admit more patients to the hospital. Conversely, fee-for-service arrangements offer no incentives to doctors to deliver the best-quality care. If a physician determines that a typical intervention for a particular problem is unnecessary, the physician is not rewarded if he doesn't perform the intervention, even though his decision saves money for the insurer and the patient. Likewise, if a physician sends a patient to a different setting where a test can be performed more efficiently, the physician does not collect a fee for making a decision that saves money.

Despite attempts at reform, medical fees in the United States are skewed to favor specialists over primary care physicians. It's no wonder that there are twice as many specialists in the United States as in Britain. Nor is it surprising that specialists in the United States perform more heart operations and do more hip replacements and give more chemotherapy than physicians in other countries. After all, physicians in the United States are paid on a fee-for-service basis.

Although American patients see more specialists, American physicians perform more procedures, and American taxpayers spend significantly more money on specialist care than their counterparts around the world, Americans are not living any longer or enjoying a better quality of life than the people in these other countries. A growing body of data shows that hospitals where patients see more physicians, get more procedures, and spend more money are not necessarily the hospitals where patients get the tests, procedures, and drugs proven to improve, lengthen, or save their lives.

Consider patients with similar illnesses in Minneapolis and Portland compared to patients in Miami. The Floridians have costs that are 2.45 times higher than those paid by the Minnesotans and the Oregonians, spend twice as many days in the hospital, are six times more likely to see specialists, and are twice as likely to end up in the intensive care unit but are slightly *less* likely to get effective medical treatments proven to extend their survival. Once again, we see a familiar pattern: cost without benefit.

Recently, a study by Dartmouth researchers showed that patients who had suffered heart attacks did no better at hospitals in which they saw more physicians. Similarly, hospitals in which patients underwent more tests and interventions were not the places where patients were *more* likely to survive after a heart attack; in fact, seeing *fewer* physicians was associated with a *higher* chance of surviving a heart attack. Spending less money was also associated with a higher chance of survival. Receiving a fee for every service encourages physicians to do more, but *more* should not be confused with *better*. Indeed, *more* frequently results in worse and more costly outcomes.

Often doctors are paid at a very low rate or not at all for crucial steps of good healthcare, such as talking with patients and coordinating their care with other physicians, nurses, and healthcare providers. Given the fee-for-service model, there is woefully little incentive for a physician working in private practice to spend time advising a diabetic patient on diet, exercise, or smoking, or to coordinate the care plan with the visiting nurse, podiatrist, ophthamologist, and family. Doctors are not paid for choosing the cheapest and most effective blood pressure pill, or for going through a patient's ten medications to figure out if they are the least costly combination. Doctors who spend too much time with patients risk going out of business in our current model of care.

Professional pride and peer recognition for a job well done, patient expectations and demands, clinical uncertainty, malpractice, and drug company blandishments can all influence physicians' decisions. Ironically, these factors tend to reinforce the fee-for-service stimulus to do more. Physicians are selected and trained to be thorough, so professional respect and peer recognition are typically awarded to physicians who consider and test for every possible condition or disease, rather than to those who are efficient and economical in how they think and test. Some physicians actually view cost considerations as a violation of the Hippocratic Oath. Direct-to-consumer advertising, Internet-fueled patient demands, and clinical uncertainty—combined with the knowledge that services will be reimbursed—often make ordering a large quantity of costly services irresistible.

We need a new American healthcare system that creates incentives to deliver the best care in the most efficient way possible, rather than a system that creates incentives to provide a wider array of services and options regardless of health benefits.

Information

Medical technology has exploded in recent years. Today, physicians can order more tests, treatments, and drugs than ever before. But the information that guides their choices has not kept pace. The FDA's drug and device evaluations often fail to compare similar drugs and devices, while drug manufacturers typically do not publish comparisons. Frequently there are no good data about the best combination of medical treatments for patients who have two or more conditions. And there are few studies about the best way to actually deliver services, such as determining the frequency with which patients should be seen in follow-up office visits and testing. To deliver the best care in the most efficient, cost-effective way, patients, physicians, and insurance companies need comparative data about different treatments that are available for the same condition. But too often those data just aren't available.

Consider treatments for early-stage prostate cancer. Until recently, reasonable options included watchful waiting, surgery, and traditional treatments of three-dimensional, conformal radiation therapy. Then came new treatments: radiation seeds implanted into the prostate (brachytherapy), intensity modulated radiation therapy (IMRT), and now proton beams. The costs for these treatments vary widely. Traditional radiation therapy costs about $11,000; the seeds run about $15,000; IMRT can cost nearly $42,500; and proton beam therapy is stratospheric. Many cancer physicians think that all of these treatments are capable of producing the same survival rates, but no one knows for sure. Nor has there been a systematic study that compares these different radiation treatments in terms of side effects such as diarrhea and impotence. Which treatment is better? This is no small question: 185,000 American men are diagnosed with prostate cancer each year, so prices that vary four-fold and more become a major economic consideration. Yet no study has compared these treatments head-to-head.

There have been some attempts to develop comparative information by conducting technology and outcomes assessments. While well-intentioned, the overall effort can charitably be described as minuscule. In 1985, the Blue Cross and Blue Shield Association established a Technology Evaluation Center, or TEC, "for assessing medical technologies through comprehensive reviews of clinical evidence." Another effort is the Drug Effectiveness Review Project, which comprises thirteen states and includes organizations eager to find evidence of a drug's safety and effectiveness and to compare it to similar drugs in the same class. The federal government's Agency for Healthcare Research and Quality also conducts some research to evaluate various medical technologies, but these efforts are seriously underfinanced. The United States spends over $2 trillion on healthcare, about $200 billion on prescription drugs, and nearly $100 billion on medical research and development of new treatments, but only a paltry $1 billion to evaluate the comparative costs and effectiveness of medical interventions and their influence on health outcomes.

A key reason for the lack of funding toward this goal is that such assessments are what economists call *public goods.* In a competitive healthcare system, private organizations have few incentives to spend money on assessments because they provide no competitive advantage to the organization, and may actually help their competitors.

The scarcity of comparative technology assessments leaves physicians with a multitude of technologies but little knowledge about their relative effectiveness. Physicians don't know if the expensive interventions are worth the cost, nor do they know how to best use combinations of interventions. It's no wonder that physicians often have a hard time determining the right thing to do, just as it's no wonder that medicine in the United States costs—and wastes—so much money.

The Institutionalization of Chaos

Every time there has been a change in how healthcare is paid for, it has been politically, strategically, and administratively easier to go along with the existing industry model of healthcare than to try to reorganize it. When the cost of healthcare was a dramatically smaller percentage of the overall economy, the method of payment was a smaller concern. However, once they were instituted, private insurance, Medicare, and Medicaid reinforced the fragmentation and fee-for-service payment system.

Before health insurance, most physicians and the American Medical Association (AMA) shunned physicians who practiced medicine in larger groups, claiming that they were replacing the family physician with faceless corporations. The AMA's hostility toward group practices extended to the health insurance industry. For years, the AMA opposed any form of healthcare insurance because they feared that insurers would try to control (doctors' medical decisions. Accordingly, employer-based) healthcare insurance was designed to mollify physicians and the AMA. The Blue Cross and Blue Shield plans, as well as plans offered by for-profit insurers, maintained the fee-for-service model and stayed far away from anything that looked like integrated, managed, or coordinated medical care. As employer-based insurance expanded, the fee-for-service payment model firmly institutionalized the centrality of the individual physician and the separate hospital. And as insurance companies became indispensable intermediaries between employers, physicians, and hospitals, they developed a vested interest in continuing the existing healthcare delivery system. Over time, these insurers have also come to feel mortally threatened by any significant reform proposal that would modify or reduce their role.

Opposition from physicians and the AMA during the enactment of Medicare and Medicaid has similarly skewed our healthcare system toward its current tangle. To neutralize the AMA and physician opposition, President Lyndon Johnson repeatedly emphasized that Medicare and Medicaid would not interfere with physicians' decision-making authority, but would only provide a neutral conduit for the money needed to pay for healthcare services. The congressional committee responsible for the Medicare and Medicaid legislation similarly emphasized that there would be no effort "to exercise control over the practice of medicine, the manner in which medical services are provided, and the administration or operation of medical facilities." There have been subsequent changes in healthcare financing, such as the HMO Act of 1973, that have encouraged employers to offer integrated health plans to their employees; but as the persistence of fragmented, fee-for-service delivery attests, these efforts were not particularly transformative. We need a new American healthcare system that creates a high-quality, efficient system rather than a fragmented, fee-for-service one.

Making Change Possible

Given the growth in healthcare costs and concerns about the quality of American healthcare, why aren't employers, Medicare, or Medicaid taking the initiative to end the fragmented, fee-for-service delivery system? Why aren't they leading the way toward facilitating coordination and integrated care? Why do the people who pay the bills seem to tolerate, if not perpetuate, this fragmented delivery system?

Unfortunately, notes Bob Galvin, director of global healthcare at General Electric, and Suzanne Delbanco, former CEO of a business-led coalition on healthcare quality called The Leapfrog Group, "Employers have largely been ineffective and unenthusiastic managers of the health benefits they sponsor." The very structure of the employer-based system actually undermines their ability to effectively control costs and improve quality.

For manufacturers of cars, computers, chemicals, and construction materials, employees' healthcare is a diversion from their primary business focus. Only a very few large companies have spent the time and resources to develop the expertise to better manage their health insurance benefits. Even fewer have made a commitment to finding ways to reform the entire healthcare system. In short, employers will do what they can to minimize premiums, but they tend not to expend resources to research and implement long-term changes to their health coverage. Fading lifetime employment reinforces this short-term focus. Given high employee turnover, employers have few incentives to invest in the long-term health of their employees. And with shorter and shorter tenure at a single company and greater pressure for quarterly profits, CEOs are less committed to their companies' long-term prospects. As a result, despite the rhetoric, only 27 percent of companies currently invest in wellness programs.

To create a market that rewards quality, efficient delivery of care, and controlled costs, employers would have to offer their employees a choice of plans and provide incentives to choose efficient, low-cost plans. Theoretically, employee demand for low-cost plans would spur insurance companies to develop networks of physicians and hospitals practicing high-quality, cost-effective medicine. Those companies capable of offering lower costs and higher quality would then be rewarded with a higher volume of patients and higher margins.

We often hear about this "market-based" healthcare system in the United States, but employer-based healthcare insurance fails in all crucial requirements for a competitive market. Its very structure virtually precludes any competition to provide high-quality, cost-effective care, leaving employers with little bargaining power. And most employees have no choice at all when it comes to their health insurance plan. Surely there is no "market" without competition and choice.

Small- and medium-sized employers that offer insurance can reasonably offer only one plan. It makes no sense for insurers to compete for business from small employers. Even larger employers rarely offer their workers choices from multiple health insurance companies. The few that do often fail to adjust the amount of the premium employees must pay if they select higher-priced insurance offerings. Furthermore, tax-deductible health insurance benefits make employees less price sensitive when they select insurance plans.

In the end, despite the hundreds of billions of dollars that employers provide for employee healthcare insurance, they have little power to drive changes in healthcare. Even corporate behemoths have little clout because their employees are spread out all over the country. In the Chicago area, Jewel-Osco food stores are the biggest employers in the region but employ fewer than 1 percent of the area's workers. Other big Chicago-based companies, including United Airlines, Abbott Laboratories, Motorola, and Walgreens, each account for fewer than 0.5 percent of the area's workers. Even in a company town like Rochester, New York, where Kodak is the largest employer, the company employs only 5 percent of all workers in the city. If large employers offer their employees multiple insurance options from several insurance companies, the employers lose even the small amount of bargaining power that their large enrollment numbers give them. Hence, except in rare instances, no single employer can provide sufficient demand to shape how medicine is delivered. As the Council for Economic Development put it:

> One or a small group of employers cannot revamp the entire system. In today's market for health insurance, there is little demand for economical care. . . . Creating competition is a collective action problem. That is, one employer offering responsible choices will not get the benefit of a reformed competitive delivery system. That takes concerted action by many employers.

Despite the tireless efforts of many well-intentioned people, the track record of forming business coalitions to have greater numbers of workers creating greater leverage for demanding more efficient healthcare options is also spotty. Coalitions require that companies develop healthcare expertise, articulate a shared vision, develop a coherent set of policies to implement their vision, and advocate their vision over time. This activity distracts businesses from Job One. More important, each step of coalition-building is problematic.

Historically, such coalitions have been fleeting, and with disappointing outcomes. Even groups that achieved notable initial success eventually failed. One of the most successful healthcare coalitions was the Pacific Business Group on Health (PBGH). To secure cheaper premiums for small businesses (two to fifty workers), it pooled businesses into a large purchasing power called PAC Advantage. In its heyday during the late 1990s, PAC Advantage offered coverage to 11,000 businesses and 147,000 Californians. But because not all businesses were required to enroll, profit-maximizing companies with younger workers sought better insurance deals outside the pool or selectively dumped their sicker and older patients into PAC Advantage. Ultimately, PAC Advantage accrued a higher number of sick, costly workers. And in order to compete with other insurers, it charged low premiums and paid insurers too little for the amount of coverage the enrollees required. Eventually, the three big insurers—Blue Shield of California, Kaiser, and Health Net—called it a day. In the summer of 2006, after thirteen years of operation, the PAC Advantage experiment in collective employer action was terminated.

Businesses have been innovating alternative approaches to managing costs and improving quality that range from tiered payments and disease management to health savings accounts, consumer-directed care, and to pay for performance. But employers are reluctantly conceding Galvin and Delbanco's pessimistic assessment of their inability to manage healthcare coverage and costs. When recently asked to rate their various strategies for reducing the growth of their health insurance costs, few businesses deemed any of them "very effective." Only one strategy, disease management, was rated as "very effective" by more than a quarter of employers. In a review of employer-based insurance, David Blumenthal, a health policy expert at Massachusetts General Hospital, summed up the problem of relying on employers to effectively address coverage, cost, and quality:

> [Healthcare] reflects the truism that "he who pays the piper calls the tune." Since business pays for a large portion of U.S. healthcare, its ability and willingness to sponsor and direct reform plays a decisive role in how the healthcare system functions. . . . Employers comprise not one tune-caller but a throng of them—increasingly diverse, lacking any legitimate conductor, and favoring a multitude of scores. . . . [Employers have] proved unable to contain the ferocious forces driving cost increases in the United States and seem to be ill-constructed to do so in the future.

Similarly, Medicaid has little clout when it comes to changing the system. Although Medicaid pays for about 15 percent of healthcare services in the United States, it offers extremely low payments to physicians and hospitals. Consequently, about half of all American physicians no longer accept Medicaid patients. For many others, Medicaid is a small, dispensable part of their practice. If Medicaid pushed too hard to change things, physicians would simply walk away.

Medicare is a somewhat different story because it controls about 30 percent of payments for healthcare in our country. It also has disproportionate influence because many insurers and employers adopt its policies regarding coverage. Recently, Medicare announced that it would cover a few unproven treatments, but only if patients were enrolled in a research trial or registry, so a determination could be made about whether or not the treatment is beneficial. Similarly, Medicare announced that it would not pay for certain preventable medical errors, such as repeat operations for leaving sponges in patients or treatments for hospital-acquired infections. Medicare is also testing some quality incentive initiatives that reward physicians and hospitals for fulfilling specific benchmarks related to heart attacks, pneumonia, and a few other conditions. Currently, Medicare administrators are thinking of paying physicians a fee for coordinating patient care.

While laudatory, these small steps hardly impact the magnitude of the problem. Medicare expects to save $20 million by refusing to pay hospitals to fix their own errors. But this constitutes roughly 0.06 percent of the money Medicare pays to hospitals each year, so there's not much of an economic incentive for hospitals to focus on error reduction. And Medicare's concept of integrated patient care is weak: Paying physicians one time for delivering a service and a second time for calling other physicians to tell them about a service hardly constitutes integrating care.

The elderly, who vote in big numbers, do not demand Medicare reform and often oppose change. Like the rest of the population, they want the freedom to go to many different physicians and hospitals. Indeed, surveys show that they equate quality with freedom of choice of physicians and hospitals. The lack of coordinated care and its impact on getting proven treatment are, to many of them, an abstraction. They do not appreciate the reality that fragmentation and fee-for-service undermine quality. Moreover, many of them don't—or can't—think about the fact that this fragmented, fee-for-service system may bankrupt the government in the future by wasting huge amounts of money on unnecessary tests and treatments today.

Other major constituencies, including physicians, hospitals, pharmaceutical companies, and insurance companies, also resist change. They spend millions of lobbying dollars to maintain the current delivery system. Resistant to and leery of government control, they are especially hostile to linking payment to anything but the number of services. Their power to maintain this model, regardless of inefficiencies, was illuminated when Congress passed the 2003 Medicare prescription drug bill, which prohibited the creation of a formulary and banned Medicare from using its buying power to negotiate lower drug prices. On an ongoing basis, even when the program reduces physician or hospital payments to control costs, Congress usually readjusts the payments a few years later when physicians and hospitals threaten to reduce patient access to care. Such seesaws remind Medicare officials that every effort to reduce costs is subject to political pushback.

When Medicare was established, it was generally understood that physicians would be paid what they charged their patients.

An assumption was made that Medicare would not consider the costs of services in determining what it covered, even though legally it has the power to do so. That is, it covers regular radiation, brachytherapy, and IMRT for prostate cancer even though the costs differ by four-fold (from $11,000 to $42,000) without any clear survival benefit and a small reduction in side effects for the extra money. Medicare hasn't used its authority to take costs into account in forty years, and it seems likely that doing so now would create a political firestorm. As the former chief medical officer at Medicare said: "By long practice, [Medicare] has not considered costs [in its coverage decisions], and has made statements in public documents saying that it does not intend to do so. This means that in order to begin considering costs, Medicare would need to go through rule-making. Politically, I think it is unlikely."

SUCH SYMPTOMS as rising numbers of uninsured Americans, exploding healthcare costs, and poor quality are the direct results of fracturing financing and delivery systems. Now forty years old, the healthcare financing system is collapsing under the burden of ever-rising costs that make it prohibitive to many Americans. A legacy of the nineteenth century, the fragmented, fee-for-service delivery system encourages physicians and hospitals to offer more procedures, ensuring increased quantity (and cost) without necessarily improving quality. For decades, efforts to reform the system have been limited to trying to fill in the cracks with the addition of a government program for individuals with chronic renal failure or for uninsured children, or to organize purchasing pools to reduce premiums for small businesses. At best, these initiatives work a bit, but they create other problems. To a large degree, the system in place prevents employers, Medicare, and Medicaid from instituting the kind of changes that can really solve problems.

We need reform. Continuing the current system, or doing nothing, would be the worst possible decision. Only comprehensive change can solve our healthcare crisis once and for all.

CHAPTER 4

The Guaranteed Healthcare Access Plan: A Comprehensive Cure

Since the passage of Medicare and Medicaid in 1965, healthcare reformers have in effect focused on rearranging the chairs on the *Titanic*, enacting cosmetic changes that ignore the system's true failures. Small changes—whether they be instituting medical savings accounts, proposing initiatives to reduce medical errors, or reforming malpractice laws—will not solve the enormous problems confronting our healthcare system. The foundations of our system are simply too old, fractured, and unstable. The only way to achieve the seven essential goals of reform is for citizens to demand comprehensive change.

The Guaranteed Healthcare Access Plan offers the simplest, most secure cure for our ailing system. Creating a new healthcare system that reconfigures 16 percent of the United States GDP is a daunting task. But the Guaranteed Healthcare Access Plan offers a public guarantee of private, high-quality healthcare. Within it, all Americans are guaranteed coverage, a choice of doctors and hospitals, and a private, accountable delivery system with the incentives to provide quality care—all at a sustainable cost. (For a summary of the Plan's ten features, see Table 4.1, below.)

TABLE 4.1 TEN FEATURES OF THE GUARANTEED HEALTHCARE ACCESS SYSTEM

FEATURES AND DESCRIPTIONS

BENEFITS AND COVERAGE

1. Guaranteed Coverage

Each American household will receive a healthcare certificate for coverage through a qualified health plan or insurance company. The certificate will *not* be a "cash card" to buy health services; rather, it is an insurance voucher entitling the individual or family to enrollment in a health plan of their choice.

2. Standard Benefits

Standard benefits will be generous, modeled on services currently received by members of Congress. Benefits include office and home visits, hospitalization, preventive screening tests, prescription drugs, some dental care, inpatient and outpatient mental-health care, and physical and occupational therapy. Patients can choose their own physicians and hospitals.

3. Freedom of Choice

With the healthcare certificate, Americans will be able to choose from among several health plans. Plans will be required to accept any enrollee without exclusions for preexisting conditions and with guaranteed renewability each year.

4. Freedom to Purchase Additional Services

Americans can use their own money to buy additional services and amenities, including a wider selection of physicians, additional mental-health benefits, coverage of complementary medicines, and "concierge medicine." Such purchases will be made with after-tax dollars.

5. Elimination of Employer-Based Insurance

The current $200 billion tax exemption for employer-based health insurance will be eliminated. Employers will stop offering health insurance, and workers' wages will rise accordingly.

6. Phasing Out of Medicare, Medicaid, and SCHIP

No one receiving benefits from Medicare, Medicaid, SCHIP, or other government programs will be forced out, but there will be no new enrollees. Current enrollees will have the option of joining the Guaranteed Healthcare Access Plan. Over a period of about fifteen years, these programs will be phased out.

OVERSIGHT AND ADMINISTRATION

7. Independent Oversight

Modeled on the Federal Reserve System, a National Health Board and twelve Regional Health Boards will be created to oversee the healthcare system. Supported by dedicated funding, the Boards will be independent of annual congressional appropriations and insulated from political and special-interest lobbying.

8. Patient Safety and Dispute Resolution

Each of the twelve Regional Health Boards will create a Center for Patient Safety and Dispute Resolution to receive and evaluate claims of injury by patients, compensate patients injured by medical error, and discipline or disqualify from practice those physicians found to be repeatedly injuring patients. Funded by a dedicated revenue, these regional Centers will develop and finance the implementation of interventions proven to enhance patient safety.

9. Cost and Quality Control

Funded through a dedicated tax, an Institute for Technology and Outcomes Assessment will assess the effectiveness and cost of new drugs, medical devices, diagnostic tests, and other interventions. It will also assess and publish the clinical outcomes of patients in the different health plans.

FINANCING

10. Dedicated Funding

Initially, the healthcare certificates will be funded by a dedicated VAT of 10 percent on purchases of goods and services. Revenue from the tax can not be diverted to other uses such as the military or Social Security. No other tax revenue will be used to pay for the Guaranteed Healthcare Access Plan. Congress has power to increase the VAT rate.

The Guaranteed Healthcare Access Plan reflects the fundamental American values of individual freedom and equality of opportunity. To realize these values, the Plan includes healthcare rights and responsibilities for both the public and private sectors. The design of this new American healthcare system maintains our government's responsibility to "promote the general welfare" by charging it with overseeing the integrity of the system and providing personal insurance certificates for all citizens, at no direct cost. (See Figure 4.1 for an overview of this Plan.) It also preserves the role of private enterprise and market incentives: The private sector—not the government—will be responsible for delivering healthcare services to all citizens, and competition with the right incentives will ensure that the providers of these services are motivated to supply high-quality care and to innovate.

FIGURE 4.1. PERSONAL HEALTHCARE VOUCHERS

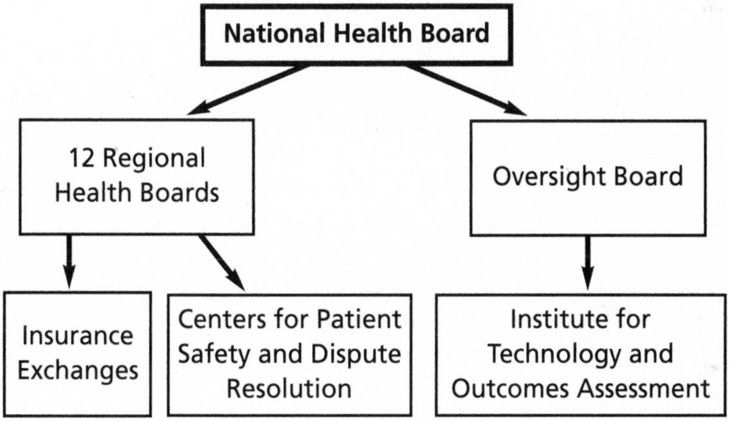

National Health Board

12 Regional Health Boards

Oversight Board

Insurance Exchanges

Centers for Patient Safety and Dispute Resolution

Institute for Technology and Outcomes Assessment

Guaranteed Coverage and Benefits

The Guaranteed Healthcare Access Plan will provide all Americans with a healthcare certificate that enables them to receive health coverage through a private insurance company or health plan. It will require no premiums or deductibles, and only minimal co-payments. Health insurance companies and plans will not be able to deny coverage to any American citizen: They will be required to enroll *anyone* who applies, and to guarantee renewal from year to year. There will be no exclusions because of preexisting health conditions.

Standard Benefits

Unlike health savings accounts, the healthcare certificate will not provide cash or a particular dollar amount for buying individual medical services. Instead, each certificate will guarantee to Americans the same benefits that members of Congress currently receive. The standard benefits will include office and home visits, hospitalization, preventive screening tests, prescription drugs, some dental care, inpatient and outpatient mental-health care, and physical and occupational therapy. This coverage is more generous than Medicare and better than that which 85 percent of Americans currently receive through their employers. The full cost of the premium will be covered by the certificate. Americans will never again have to worry about unaffordable health insurance.

Choice

Each year Americans will be notified of their entitlement to a healthcare certificate, which they can use to enroll in any government-approved health insurance company or other provider organization in an "Insurance Exchange." Individuals and families—not government and not their employer—will choose which plan they want to enroll in. In most regions, consumers will have a choice among five to eight qualified health plans or insurance companies. In larger cities, as many as fifteen or twenty competing plans might exist; in rural areas there might be only one or two plans. Charts from one of the twelve Regional Health Boards (again, see Figure 4.1) will identify the similarities and differences in the services offered by the competing health insurance providers, including their regional networks of participating physicians and hospitals, their list of co-payments, and so on. People who have private coverage today will be able to keep their physicians, and most aspects of their plans will remain unchanged.

Under the Guaranteed Healthcare Access Plan, Americans will be free to purchase health coverage for additional services or amenities not included among the standard health benefits. For a fee, individuals can purchase a greater choice of physicians and hospitals, access to a greater variety of drugs, more mental-health benefits, complementary and alternative medicines, experimental interventions for serious conditions, and "concierge medicine" packages that eliminate waiting times for office visits and allow physicians to make house calls. Payments for any additional coverage would not be tax deductible.

Delivery of Care

After the individual has decided on a plan, the chosen company will then implement the policy and manage the delivery of healthcare services through its network of physicians and hospitals. To qualify for participation in an Insurance Exchange, health plans and insurance companies must agree to provide the standard set of benefits for the value of the healthcare certificate. Qualified health insurance companies and plans will be otherwise largely free to structure their businesses as they see fit. They will be able to shrink or expand their physician and hospital networks to attract certificate holders, offer different drug formularies, more disease management programs, a particular choice of specialists, and a range of specialty hospitals. These health insurance companies and plans might even offer benefits not covered by the healthcare certificate, at no additional charge. Other than co-payments, the insurance providers will *not* be able to charge certificate holders for coverage of standard benefits.

The health insurance companies and health plans will be reimbursed with a risk-adjusted premium for each individual or family enrolling with a certificate. This payment will be adjusted for age, sex, smoking status, preexisting conditions, and other factors, as determined by the National Health Board (as further discussed below). Such an adjustment will eliminate the incentive for insurance companies to "cherry pick"—that is, to avoid sicker patients and enroll only young, healthy ones.

Implementation

Initially, the Guaranteed Healthcare Access Plan will cover the 177 million Americans who are not covered by Medicare, Medicaid, SCHIP, or another government healthcare program. Americans whose healthcare is currently paid through these programs will have the choice to keep their current coverage or switch to the Guaranteed Healthcare Access Plan. No one receiving benefits from Medicare, Medicaid, SCHIP, or other government health programs will be forced out. The 44 million Americans enrolled in Medicare and the 36 million Americans who receive Medicaid, SCHIP, and other government health benefits will be notified that they have a choice: They can either remain in their government-funded program or join the Guaranteed Healthcare Access Plan.

After the Guaranteed Healthcare Access Plan is established, no new enrollees will be allowed in Medicare, Medicaid, SCHIP, or other current government programs. People now receiving Medicaid or SCHIP will switch permanently to the new plan if they became ineligible for their current program. Americans turning 65 after the Guaranteed Healthcare Access Plan goes into effect will just remain in it. In less than fifteen years from implementation, *all* Americans regardless of age, income, employment, health, or marital status will receive the same standard benefits within one healthcare system.

Efficient Oversight and Administration

The current healthcare system is so complex that no single person understands all of its inner workings. Responsibility for administration, regulation, and oversight is divided among thousands of organizations, and yet many important issues, such as patient safety, are unmonitored and unregulated by any official body. The

Guaranteed Healthcare Access Plan will solve the inefficiencies of administration that currently hamper our healthcare system. Through a unique oversight and administrative structure, the voucher system will accomplish the goals of comprehensive reform and provide durable checks and balances.

A National Health Board with twelve Regional Health Boards, modeled on the Federal Reserve System, will oversee the system and control costs. To reduce political interference and allow the necessary tough choices to be made, members of these Boards will be nominated by the president and confirmed by the Senate for fixed, long, and staggered terms, which can be renewed only once. To further ensure objectivity and independence from political pressure and special-interest influence peddling, funding for its administration would come from dedicated money rather than from annual congressional appropriations.

Specifically, the National Health Board will be responsible for:

- defining and regularly adjusting the standard health benefits covered by the healthcare certificate to reflect changes in standards of care, advances in technology, and fiscal realities.
- conducting research to determine the risk adjustments necessary for premiums paid to healthcare insurers and plans.
- determining payment based on regional differences in cost of living.

- sponsoring research on quality, outcomes, and performance of the healthcare system.
- overseeing and coordinating the Regional Health Boards.
- reporting regularly to Congress and the American public on their healthcare system.

For their part, the twelve Regional Health Boards will be responsible for:

- organizing and overseeing the Insurance Exchanges.
- certifying that each private health insurance company and health plan in an Insurance Exchange has a sufficient network of hospitals and physicians and adequate financial reserves, and that the plan or insurer is in fact providing the standard benefits to all enrollees.
- managing the enrollment of individuals and families in health insurance companies and health plans.
- assigning coverage to Americans who do not enroll on their own.
- overseeing the regional Centers for Patient Safety and Dispute Resolution.

Each quarter, insurance companies will provide aggregate data to Regional Health Boards on their performance, including patient satisfaction, disenrollment rates, use of preventive services such as mammograms and Pap smears, hospitalization, mortality rates, and patient outcomes for various conditions. With these data, the Regional Health Boards will analyze, monitor, and disseminate information on the quality of healthcare delivered by individual insurance companies.

Malpractice Reform

Each Regional Health Board will have a Center for Patient Safety and Dispute Resolution staffed by patients, physicians, and lawyers to remedy the ills of our current malpractice system. These Centers will be responsible for

- receiving and adjudicating patient complaints about medical errors and injuries.
- compensating patients whose injuries were caused by medical error.
- disciplining and disqualifying those physicians and health professionals repeatedly responsible for injuring patients or violating established safety procedures.
- developing and funding the implementation of proven patient-safety interventions in health plans, hospitals, physicians' office, pharmacies, and other provider sites.

Patients not satisfied by a Center's resolution of their complaint would still be able to sue for malpractice.

Monitoring Quality

Finally, to control healthcare inflation and to monitor the performance of insurance companies and health plans, an Institute for Technology Outcomes and Assessment will be established. The Institute will be responsible for:

- systematically reviewing research studies and data on the effectiveness and cost of various drugs, devices, diagnostic tests, and new technologies.
- sponsoring research studies to compare those interventions for which data are currently lacking.
- collecting data from health plans and insurance companies on patient outcomes and on the drugs, medical technologies, and interventions used.
- disseminating data on drugs, devices, and other technologies and outcomes to health plans, physicians, patients, drug and technology manufacturers, and the general public.

The Institute's operations will be overseen by an independent board appointed by the National Health Board.

A Better Financing System

Most people suspect that covering all Americans will require adding tens, if not hundreds, of billions of dollars to the healthcare system. But the cost of the Guaranteed Healthcare Access Plan will *not* exceed the amount now being spent on healthcare. The healthcare system does not need *more* money—it needs to spend money more efficiently. More important, healthcare spending cannot be permitted to suck money from every other national program. Instead, it must reflect the growth of the economy and the public's willingness and ability to pay for healthcare services. The Guaranteed Healthcare Access Plan has multiple built-in mechanisms for keeping costs down over time and making healthcare reform sustainable.

All workers who now receive healthcare coverage through their employers—whether they work in a factory, an office, or a government agency—will see more money in their paychecks with the Guaranteed Healthcare Access Plan. Americans will no longer have to pay premiums or deductibles. The portion of the premiums for their health insurance that employers provide will come back to Americans as a pay raise. Because so-called fringe benefits, like healthcare coverage, are just another form of compensation, the money that employers were spending on healthcare coverage will be paid, instead, to employees in the form of higher salaries. Employers often prevent their employees from accepting job offers from competitors by supplying substantial benefits. Without the issue of healthcare coverage, employers will entice employees to stay with—or to join—their company by offering higher salaries. (The amount of increase will depend primarily on the amount of money previously spent on employee health insurance. According to the Census Bureau, the range is between 7 percent and 14 percent, with an average of 8.5 percent.)

As state and local governments stop paying for Medicaid, SCHIP, insurance for state employees, hospital supplements, and many other health expenses (which now account for about a third of state budgets), state budgets—and thus income, sales, and other taxes—will drop substantially. Eventually, there will be no payroll deductions for Medicare. In addition, most of the $300 billion the federal government now spends for healthcare beyond the money that comes from the Medicare tax will be eliminated. The additional income that employees receive in their paychecks and the lower federal and state taxes are big financial benefits associated with the Guaranteed Healthcare Access Plan.

Instead of the myriad premiums, taxes, and other payments that currently fund healthcare, the Guaranteed Healthcare Access Plan will be paid for by a *dedicated* value-added tax, or VAT. It is similar to a sales tax on purchases of goods and services. The VAT ensures that *all* Americans will contribute money to the healthcare system. Like taxes for Social Security, Medicare, or the highway trust fund, the VAT is dedicated—it cannot be diverted to *any* other purpose, including spending for the military, college loans, Social Security, or air traffic control improvements. Because only money raised by the VAT will support the Guaranteed Healthcare Access Plan, the rate of the VAT and the level of coverage included in the standard set of benefits will be directly correlated: The more generous the benefits offered, the higher the tax rate. To cover the 257 million Americans not receiving Medicare, the rate will be about 10 percent.

In 2006, the annual premium for the high-end Blue Cross/Blue Shield preferred-provider plan available to members of Congress—the standard benefits plan used as the model for coverage under the Guaranteed Healthcare Access Plan—was $5,180 for individuals and $11,216 for families. At these rates, insuring all 257 million Americans not covered by Medicare would cost a total of $944.7 billion.

But the cost of providing coverage for all Americans cannot be derived from such a simple multiplication process. Although some uninsured Americans are relatively healthy (children, workers, and young "invincibles"), others are unhealthy and covering them will make costs rise. The Medicaid population, who tend to be sicker than average federal employees, would cost even more. Based on calculations by the Urban Institute, the estimated cost of including these Americans in the Guaranteed Healthcare Access Plan would increase the total cost by about $50 billion. Adjusting the premiums of Congress's plan being used as a reference to reflect this greater use of services would require $994.7 billion to cover all 257 million Americans not currently covered by Medicare.

How does this compare with current healthcare spending? Excluding what was spent on nursing-home care, federal and state governments spent $261 billion on Medicaid alone in 2006 (see Table 4.2). That same year, the nation's total expenditure for private health insurance—not including out-of-pocket expenses for prescriptions, dental services, and other healthcare expenses—was $723 billion. Furthermore, at least $10 billion was spent on subsidizing hospitals, maternal and child care, and other programs that are needed for the safety net for the uninsured. (This does not include the billions spent for the Indian Health Service, the Defense Department, or veterans' health benefits.) Altogether in 2006, the United States spent roughly $1002 billion on healthcare for those Americans not enrolled in Medicare.

TABLE 4.2. CURRENT HEALTHCARE SPENDING*

Program	Total Annual Costs
Employer-based private insurance	$723 billion
Medicaid and SCHIP	$269 billion
Other programs— hospital subsidies, maternal and child care, etc.	$10 billion
Total non-Medicare	**$1002 billion**

*All calculations in Tables 4.2 and 4.3 are in 2006 dollars because that is the last year the government has tallied costs in the current healthcare system.

The Guaranteed Healthcare Access Plan will end up saving us a great deal of money (see Table 4.3). Administrative costs will be significantly lower as underwriting, sales, and marketing costs for insurance companies drop. Byzantine determinations of eligibility or income for subsidies for particular government programs will cease to exist. State costs for administering Medicaid and SCHIP will be eliminated. These administrative savings alone would constitute about $70 to $100 billion. And because employers will no longer need such large human resource departments to manage health benefits, track health contributions, or hire consultants to evaluate various insurance options, they, too, will save billions of dollars. Nor will citizens waste productive time gathering data for means testing.

Although administrative savings reflect one-time savings, the lower overall cost of the Guaranteed Healthcare Access Plan will offer coverage to all Americans without increasing the total

TABLE 4.3. THE ECONOMICS OF THE GUARANTEED HEALTHCARE ACCESS PLAN

Group	Number of Americans	Average Premium	Total Annual Costs
Individuals	41.2 million	$5,180	$213.4 billion
Families	65.2 million	$11,216	$731.3 billion
Total for non-Medicare population	257 million		$944.7 billion
Adjustment for greater healthcare needed by uninsured and Medicaid populations			$50 billion*
Total non-Medicare costs	**257 million**		**$995 billion**

*About 25 percent of Americans under 65 are uninsured or in Medicaid and SCHIP. According to estimates, they are sicker than average and likely to use about 26 percent more healthcare services than average. In short, covering them would increase costs about $50 billion.

national healthcare spending. All the money needed to cover healthcare would be generated by the VAT. In the end, the total cost will equal our current costs, but with far wider coverage and a more efficient overall system.

The key to a sustainable healthcare plan is establishing built-in mechanisms to keep the rate of cost increases down. The rate of increase in healthcare spending over time cannot continue as it has for the last few decades, at a rate 2.1 percent faster than that of our GDP. With the Guaranteed Healthcare Access Plan, a cost-control "rheostat" will ensure that all healthcare expenditures and revenues will be explicitly connected through the dedicated VAT. If Americans want more money for healthcare services, they will have to persuade Congress to increase the VAT levy. Americans' aversion to tax increases will restrain demands unless the added healthcare services are considered worth the cost.

The Guaranteed Healthcare Access Plan incorporates four other mechanisms for effective, long-term cost controls that counter the current counterproductive government price controls and centralized management of local spending. Competition among health insurance companies and plans will restrain costs. Since health plans and insurance companies will have the same risk-adjusted, fixed payment per enrollee for a standard set of benefits—and have to guarantee enrollment and renewal—they will compete for members, and will have increased incentive to be efficient. Such competition will most likely generate innovations in the management of chronic illnesses, which currently commands 70 percent of healthcare spending. Because of the exorbitant cost of hospitalization, health plans will need to develop ways to keep patients with chronic conditions healthier. They will need to limit spending on technology that offers little or no health improvements, and eliminate duplicate testing by different doctors. And health plans and insurance companies will need to experiment with how to reimburse physicians, hospitals, and other providers to coordinate their care and deliver it in the most efficient setting.

Second, because Americans who want to purchase additional health insurance benefits will have to pay extra with after-tax dollars, they will have an incentive to spend judiciously to receive value for their money. This will help keep costs in check.

In an effort to ensure efficiency, the Institute for Technology and Outcomes Assessment will evaluate the effectiveness, cost, and value of new and existing drugs, devices, and other kinds of technologies. The Institute will also identify and promote procedures that save money without reducing quality of care. Such data will provide vital information for health plans and insurance companies as they design more efficient and effective care, and the work of the Institute will help detect any cost cutting that harms patients.

The Institute's research will help health plan administrators and health insurance companies to cover cost-effective, proven care with less fear of litigation. Indeed, doctors today may order unnecessary tests because they fear lawsuits. The new Centers for Patient Safety and Dispute Resolution will consider the Institute's evaluations to be informed medical decisions that allow for a "safe harbor" for the actual implementation of cost-effective care by health plans.

Finally, the Institute's assessments will change the dynamics of long-term medical research and development. In particular, its decisions will encourage drug and medical-device companies to focus their research and development on high-value interventions. Today, these companies develop new interventions with little regard for price or the degree of improvement over existing interventions. By providing more reliable information on future coverage decisions, and by emphasizing cost-effectiveness, the independent Institute will help shift research priorities toward technologies that provide real improvements in survival and health. In this new scenario, no amount of advertising razzle-dazzle could create broad, profitable markets for them. Other companies will begin to focus their attention on developing products, processes, and procedures that improve care delivery and coordination to improve quality and reduce costs.

No single cost-control mechanism is likely to be effective in restraining the rise in healthcare expenditures. But together, these different mechanisms pulling in the same direction should make a difference.

The Seven Goals of Reform

1. Guaranteed Coverage

Under the Guaranteed Healthcare Access Plan, all Americans—100 percent of them—will have private health insurance coverage. There will be no cracks—no eligibility requirements based on income or employment—through which people can fall. Americans will be guaranteed healthcare coverage whether they are employed in a dream job, are starting their own companies, or have a child with cancer or a preexisting condition. No one will need to worry about being denied coverage or renewal because of a family illness, nor will anyone be threatened by unaffordable insurance premiums. In an era of global competition, outsourcing, downsizing, and general uncertainty, this

Guaranteed Healthcare Access Plan offers healthcare security to Americans nationwide.

For Americans who get health insurance through their employer, the Guaranteed Healthcare Access Plan will be easy and straightforward. Just as they get information on their options from their employer, they will be informed by their Regional Health Board about what insurance companies are available and how to enroll. For the self-insured, those who receive Medicaid, and the uninsured, the Guaranteed Healthcare Access Plan will offer up a simple solution to coverage. They will no longer be required to get quotes from insurance brokers, go through insurance physicals, or bring armfuls of documents to a Medicaid office. Best of all, if people forget to enroll or something goes wrong with their enrollment, they won't be left out: The Regional Health Board will automatically enroll them in an insurance plan with the same standard benefits.

2. Effective Cost Controls

The Guaranteed Healthcare Access Plan is the only reform plan with credible cost controls. Most of the administrative overhead of the current insurance system will be eliminated. With large Insurance Exchanges and the pooling of millions of Americans, the underwriting, sales, and marketing that currently exist will cease. The jumble of current government programs—each with its own bureaucracy, rules, regulations, and operating procedures—will no longer exist. The Guaranteed

Healthcare Access Plan will do away with means testing; our government won't have to waste inordinate amounts of time and money to determine who is or is not eligible for federal programs, such as with Medicaid or SCHIP. As an added benefit, the humiliation associated with means testing will become a thing of the past.

Over time, five different cost-control levers will restrain costs: competition among health plans to provide the same benefits at lower cost and higher quality; the demand for value when Americans purchase additional services; the evaluation of effectiveness and cost of new technologies covered by the benefits package; new incentives for drug and other medical technology companies; and a dedicated VAT that limits health cost increases. This combination of forces allows for innovation while keeping the Guaranteed Healthcare Access Plan fiscally sustainable.

3. High-Quality, Coordinated Care

The Guaranteed Healthcare Access Plan provides health insurance companies and plans with strong incentives to implement the three *I*'s of quality coordinated care: infrastructure, information, and incentives. With Regional Health Boards collecting outcomes information and demanding accountability from companies that participate in the Insurance Exchanges, there will be strong motivation to create an efficient infrastructure, deliver coordinated healthcare services, reduce medical errors, and establish electronic medical records systems. The National Health Board, for instance, will not micro-manage health plan administrators; it will not tell them which electronic medical record to install. Instead, it will simply require that they have interoperability and regularly provide data on how well their patients are doing. Health insurance companies and plans will be hard-pressed to deliver the required data without electronic medical records that reach across physicians, hospitals, and other providers. Furthermore, to ensure that their outcomes are good, insurance companies will have to organize care more effectively. Under the Guaranteed Healthcare Access Plan, patients with diabetes, emphysema, high blood pressure, and other chronic conditions will probably receive home visits from nurses, telephone calls, and reminders to monitor diet, medications, and vaccines. Health insurance companies and plans might eliminate co-payments for essential medications to encourage patients with chronic conditions to take medications regularly. And patients with minor complaints may receive preemptive appointments for treatment and instruction in preventive measures.

Furthermore, prevention and wellness will be boosted. As demonstrated in other countries, health plans and insurance companies will most likely retain the same enrollees for years. Healthy individuals will have more proactive contacts with healthcare providers to obtain screening tests, vaccinations, exercise recommendations, and smoking cessation programs. Health plans and insurance companies might develop novel collaborations with schools, companies, and others to combat the obesity epidemic because they themselves will be saddled with the costs of increasing weight.

By disseminating comparative information and providing citizens with choices of health insurance providers, the Guaranteed Healthcare Access Plan will enable Americans to participate in the system as informed consumers. Informed decision making and choice are requirements of any true market—and, indeed, the Guaranteed Healthcare Access Plan sets the stage for free enterprise to deliver on its promise that competition will drive quality up while driving prices down.

Giving insurance companies and health plans an opportunity to compare their performance with that of other organizations in the Insurance Exchanges will stimulate improvement, which, in turn, will most likely encourage the coordination and integration of care. Health plans and insurance companies will also be motivated to craft their financial reimbursements so that physicians and other providers implement patient safety measures and follow best practices. Thus the Guaranteed Healthcare Access Plan will motivate the health insurance companies and plans to innovate in finding ways to deliver quality, coordinated care.

By making the private sector accountable for delivery of healthcare services and the public sector responsible for funding and oversight, the Guaranteed Healthcare Access Plan creates an environment that generates high-quality, coordinated care for the public good while also supporting private enterprise.

One of the most shameful and unjust aspects of the current healthcare system in the United States is the way health insurance companies attempt to sign up young, healthy people while avoiding the sick—the very people who need coverage. Some people worry that relying on private health plans and insurance companies will produce the same behavior. The Guaranteed Healthcare Access Plan will block such discrimination—in part, by requiring all health insurance companies and plans to offer the standard set of benefits requiring guaranteed enrollment and annual renewal. But its ultimate safeguard against such tactics is *risk adjustment*—changing how much is paid to insurance companies for factors such as age, sex, smoking status, and preexisting conditions. The Regional Health Boards will pay health insurance companies and plans more money per patient on average when the organizations enroll older, sicker patients, and less money when they enroll young, healthy people.

Admittedly, risk adjustment is an imperfect science, and the National Health Board will need to conduct research on improving it. Fortunately, some healthcare plans in the United States, as well as health authorities in countries such as the Netherlands and Israel, have relevant experience that will undoubtedly prove helpful to the National Health Board. In the meantime, America's healthcare system could institute a form of reinsurance. (For instance, Regional Health Boards might pick up the excess when costs rise above $100,000 for a single patient.)

4. Choice

Through the Insurance Exchanges, Americans will be able to choose a health insurance company or plan providing the standard set of healthcare benefits. Because of guaranteed enrollment and renewability every year without consideration of past medical histories, the choice of plan will be ours. No American can be turned away, rejected, discontinued, or face sky-high premiums. All Americans will have the choice to purchase additional health coverage for services or amenities that are not part of the standard health benefits.

5. Fair Funding

In the ongoing arguments about establishing a healthcare system that guarantees coverage for all Americans, citizens consistently demand fair funding. We want a plan that requires all people to pay into the system. Recalling their introductory economics class, some Americans bemoan the idea of a national VAT to pay for health coverage, seeing it as regressive and unfair. Although this contention is widely repeated, it is simplistic at best. The fairness of any proposal cannot be properly evaluated by considering the tax alone. The benefits funded by the tax must also be considered—in addition to the costs and benefits of alternative policies, and the cost of doing nothing at all.

The current healthcare system in the United States is heavily biased in favor of the rich who receive a substantially bigger tax break for healthcare coverage—about *four times* that of the working poor. Under the Guaranteed Healthcare Access Plan, all Americans will pay the VAT in proportion to their consumption.

Poorer Americans—as well as all of those who are sick and therefore need more healthcare services—would generally receive much more in benefits than they would pay in the VAT. Health coverage for a family today costs over $12,000 a year. In the Guaranteed Healthcare Access Plan, anyone earning less than the median income will pay less than $4,500 per year. The value of the health coverage that poorer individuals and families will receive under the Guaranteed Healthcare Access Plan greatly exceeds what they pay in tax for coverage. This fair and reasonable system of payment is the hallmark of progressivity.

6. Reasonable Dispute Resolution

There is no doubt that comprehensive healthcare reform requires a monumental change to the current malpractice system, which not only hurts both doctors and patients but also is far too expensive. The Guaranteed Healthcare Access Plan addresses the malpractice mess by creating Centers for Patient Safety and Dispute Resolution in each geographic region. The Centers will pay for initial investigation, adjudication, and compensation of claims, so physicians will not have to pay malpractice premiums at current levels. Healthcare providers might want to retain malpractice insurance for protection if dissatisfied patients elect to sue after a hearing at their Center, but only a small amount of such insurance should be necessary. Patients who have been harmed, for their part, will receive fair compensation much more quickly.

7. *Economic Revitalization*

Aside from its obvious improvements to the nation's health, the Guaranteed Healthcare Access Plan will sever the link between employment and health insurance and restrain the growth in healthcare costs. Removing ongoing responsibilities and obligations for employee and retiree healthcare coverage from the list of company responsibilities will reduce the financial and administrative burdens of managing employee health insurance—thus making businesses more efficient and competitive.

By reducing the spending on human resource departments and the consultants required to manage healthcare benefits for employees, businesses will free up money to increase wages and invest in core business priorities. Free of the unpredictability of future healthcare cost increases, employers will once again be able to base hiring decisions on business goals and productivity rather than on future healthcare costs and fringe benefit rates. Over time, this realignment of priorities should boost employment.

Workers win, too. Under the Guaranteed Healthcare Access Plan, employees will demand and receive higher wages since they will no longer be getting healthcare benefits from their employers. Strikes and tough negotiations over health give-backs will become less frequent because healthcare benefits will not be tied to compensation. And the fear of losing healthcare insurance will no longer compel workers to stay in jobs where they are no longer happy or productive. Instead, employees will be more able to change jobs and start new enterprises.

By severing the tie between employment and healthcare insurance, the Guaranteed Healthcare Access Plan will result in a boost of approximately $200 billion in federal income tax revenues with the elimination of the tax benefit for employer-based health insurance. The compensation that was previously awarded to employees as untaxed healthcare benefits will be distributed instead as wages. Some employers might still provide extended coverage for healthcare services not included in the standard benefits as a fringe benefit to attract or reward workers, but these added benefits would be taxed like other compensation, rather than being exempt from tax as employer-provided health benefits are today.

Table 4.4, below, provides a succinct list of these proposed healthcare goals.

TABLE 4.4. GUARANTEED HEALTHCARE ACCESS AND THE GOALS OF REFORM

GOALS, QUESTIONS, AND ANSWERS FOR THE GUARANTEED HEALTHCARE ACCESS PLAN

1. Guaranteed Coverage

Does the proposal for a new American healthcare system guarantee healthcare coverage for all Americans—not 96 percent or 97 percent, but 100 percent? Does the proposal guarantee a defined set of benefits that includes office and home visits, hospitalization, preventive screening tests, prescription drugs, some dental care, mental-health care, and physical and occupational therapies, with no deductibles and minimal co-payments?

YES. The Guaranteed Healthcare Access Plan guarantees healthcare coverage for 100 percent of Americans. There are no cracks. All citizens will receive the same benefits that members of Congress do, including office and home visits, hospitalization, preventive screening tests, prescription drugs, some dental care, mental-health care, and physical and occupational therapies. There are no premiums or deductibles. There is guaranteed enrollment and renewability and there are no exclusions for preexisting conditions. Americans who fail to sign up for a health plan will be covered.

2. Effective Cost Controls

Does the proposal improve efficiency by reducing excessive administrative costs and reducing fraud? Does the proposal eliminate multiple financing mechanisms and redundant bureaucracies? Will the proposal rein in rising costs of healthcare inflation from diffusion of technology and cost-ineffective care?

YES. The system will be much more efficient. There will be a significant reduction of insurance underwriting, sales, and marketing costs; elimination of means testing to determine eligibility and subsidies for government programs. Fixed payment for the standard benefits will produce incentives for health plans and insurance companies to deliver care efficiently. Five long-term cost-control mechanisms will operate: (1) A dedicated VAT will limit what can be spent each year on healthcare. (2) Competition between health plans will restrain costs. (3) Americans who buy additional services with their own after-tax money will be cost-conscious. (4) The Institute for Technology and Outcomes Assessment will provide information on effectiveness and cost to eliminate tests and treatments of marginal or no value. (5) Systematic technology assessments will shift R&D by drug and medical-device companies toward more cost-effective interventions.

3. High-Quality, Coordinated Care

Does the reform proposal have a mechanism to reduce medical errors, hospital-acquired infections, and high-cost/low-to-no-benefit treatments? Does the proposal encourage coordinated care and innovation in delivery, while also holding providers accountable for high-quality health outcomes? Is there a process for regularly evaluating the quality of these providers?

YES. The system makes health insurers and plans accountable for quality. They must report outcomes quarterly to Regional Health Boards. Public reporting of the data will encourage investment in infrastructure, information technology, and the integration of care delivery. The Institute for Technology Outcomes and Assessment will conduct research and disseminate information that will improve quality. The Center for Patient Safety and Dispute Resolution will promote and fund proven patient safety interventions.

4. Choice

Will Americans be able to choose their health insurance plans, physicians, and hospitals? Does the proposal give citizens the freedom to purchase extra healthcare benefits beyond the standard benefits guaranteed to all?

YES. Americans can choose a health insurance plan that includes their current doctors and hospitals. Americans can also choose to purchase additional healthcare services beyond the standard set of benefits provided by the certificate.

5. Fair Funding

Does the proposal have financing in which all Americans contribute fairly?

YES. By eliminating employer-based health insurance, workers will see an increase in wages. By phasing out Medicare, Medicaid, and

SCHIP, Americans will experience a reduction in federal and state taxes. All Americans will pay a dedicated VAT on purchases, and all Americans will receive the same healthcare coverage. For an average American family with the median income, the value of the healthcare certificate will be over $12,000 and the payment in VAT will be under $4,500.

6. Reasonable Dispute Resolution

Does the new healthcare system proposal offer a mechanism for rational dispute resolution that quickly and efficiently compensates patients who are harmed while at the same time protecting physicians from frivolous lawsuits and skyrocketing malpractice premiums?

YES. Each state or region will have a Center for Patient Safety and Dispute Resolution that will evaluate, resolve, and, if appropriate, compensate patients for medical injuries. Citizens who are dissatisfied with a Center's decision about a claim will be able to file a lawsuit privately. Physicians will be able to have minimal or no malpractice insurance.

7. Economic Revitalization

Does the proposal eliminate healthcare considerations from the purview of business, so businesses can focus on the core competencies? Will the new system guarantee total insurance portability? Will the proposal reduce labor-management conflict and permit hiring based on productivity and not fringe benefits?

YES. The link between healthcare and employment will be severed, freeing employers to increase wages and make other investments. Employers will make hiring decisions based on productivity rather than in terms of the impact on outlays for fringe benefits. Workers will receive pay increases and be freed from job-lock. Labor-management conflict will be reduced.

Secret Features of the Guaranteed Healthcare Access Plan

Beyond the seven goals discussed above, two of the most significant features of the Guaranteed Healthcare Access Plan are implicit: It is comparatively simple and it coheres with fundamental American values.

Nothing that changes the way almost $1 out of every $6 is raised and spent in an economy can be entirely simple, but the Guaranteed Healthcare Access Plan has relatively few moving parts. It envisages one standard set of benefits for all Americans without income-linked subsidies and contains none of the complex administration that means testing requires. It relies on one funding source, the VAT, rather than on many different streams including employer contributions, worker premiums, deductibles, Medicare taxes, and other state and federal taxes. With one Insurance Exchange per region, the number of health plans and insurance companies nationwide will be substantially reduced and employers will be freed of responsibility for providing healthcare. Administration will be handled by one National Health Board and twelve Regional Health Boards. In short, the Guaranteed Healthcare Access Plan replaces the confusing, contradictory, and counterproductive incentives that insurance companies, physicians, and hospitals now receive with clear, effective signals.

The Plan's single biggest advantage is its accurate reflection of quintessential American values: equality of opportunity and individual freedom. As Tocqueville noted, the United States differs from many other Western countries in that it emphasizes an egalitarian ethos premised not on equal outcomes but on equal opportunity. The Guaranteed Healthcare Access Plan will offer everyone the same standard benefits, funded by a tax that everyone pays. At the same time, the new system lets individual freedom flourish. Competition among insurance companies will improve quality, efficiency, and innovation in delivering services from physicians and hospitals. And the Guaranteed Healthcare Access Plan will give Americans a choice of health plans, physicians, and hospitals operating in the private sector and the option to buy more coverage for amenities and a wider range of services.

THE GUARANTEED HEALTHCARE ACCESS PLAN is the best policy alternative to establish a sustainable healthcare system. It gives all Americans the security of seamless, continuous, lifelong coverage. The peace of mind engendered by this safety net is beyond economic analysis. It is priceless.

CHAPTER 5

Band-Aids Are Not Enough

At what point does a cruise line invest in a new ship instead of once again patching up a rusty hull? When does an airline decide that a passenger jet is getting too old to repair? When do we stop sending our kids to school on old buses and decide to order new ones? The answer: When the risk of not biting the bullet puts lives at stake.

It's not easy to make big changes, particularly when it involves altering years of established systems or behaviors. There is no doubt that implementing a new healthcare system for America will be very demanding. Some people do not think it can be done; it's too difficult, they say. Some professional policy advocates argue that Americans prefer evolutionary, incremental change over comprehensive reform. But we are smart enough to know when something is beyond repair—and, indeed, most Americans have accepted the fact that our healthcare system has reached the point of no return.

We certainly need comprehensive reform. Other than the Guaranteed Healthcare Access Plan, no proposal for comprehensive reform has been offered up that reflects our nation's core values by providing for government guarantee of quality private healthcare. Our alternative has been to limp along, opting for smaller, incremental reforms and trying things out to see what might work.

A champion of this "try-it-on-for-size" approach is Stuart Butler, a health policy expert at the conservative Heritage Foundation think tank who rejects the possibility for large-scale change to our current system:

> I think that strategies based on large changes for people, particularly people who currently have [health] coverage, will fail. I think that is one of the lessons of the Clinton plan. . . . It is far better to make minimal changes—important but minimal changes—to those parts of the system that work tolerably well. . . . [I]t is very important to recognize that we are likely to see significant improvements come from continuous experimentation, not by centralized, government decisions.
>
> It makes sense to try different approaches, and the ones that succeed will tend to eventually crowd out the ones that are less successful. I think that's the only way to find out the right answer to this. The alternative is to say, let's try to figure it all out in Washington and impose it everywhere and just hope we pick the right solution. One of the problems of nationalizing this is that with the Congress making these decisions you seem to freeze progress pretty rapidly.

Butler's is not just a standard conservative, small-government view. It has bipartisan support. Kenneth Thorpe, a health policy professor at Emory University who was heavily involved in

President Bill Clinton's healthcare reform effort, argues that "President Bill Clinton's ambitious and far-reaching Health Security Act . . . would have provided universal coverage, while redesigning the financing, structure, and provision of health care. It was the scope and reach of the Clinton proposal that proved to be its downfall."

There are many reasons people support incremental reform. Some prefer to test out reform ideas before widely implementing them; others seek to benefit from particular reforms. Purveyors of information technology, for instance, are enthusiastic about subsidies to physicians and hospitals for installing electronic medical records. Financial institutions support medical savings accounts that will give them another source of revenue. Others, particularly politicians and professional policy advocates who have become frustrated by futile fights for comprehensive healthcare reform, have concluded that "half a loaf is better than nothing." They give up on comprehensive reform, believing that incremental changes have a better chance of being enacted. And the status quo is preferred by businesses involved in healthcare that are making handsome profits from the current system. To stave off major reform or create interest-group paralysis, however, they too are willing to support incremental changes.

The Many Flavors of Incremental Reform

Incremental "reform" in healthcare is not a new concept. Indeed, it is not really "reform" at all, but just maintenance, which is exactly what we've been doing for the last forty years. It's like taking an old computer in for service, repairs, or upgrades: We've been patching up and adding on to the same old system.

Since the enactment of Medicare and Medicaid in 1965, many "minimal changes" have made an appearance: In the 1970s, we extended Medicare to include people with chronic renal failure. In the 1980s, we changed Medicare's formulae for paying physicians and hospitals to hold down costs. In the 1990s, we established SCHIP to offer coverage to more children. In 2003, Congress enacted a drug benefit in Medicare. We introduced tiered drug formularies and health savings accounts as an attempt to keep medical costs down and changed malpractice laws to reduce defensive medicine.

But what have all these incremental changes produced? Are we better off today than we were forty years ago? Have innovative approaches crowded out the less successful ones to create an improved healthcare system, as the Heritage Foundation's Stuart Butler predicted they would? If these measures had significantly improved the system, citizens would be largely satisfied with healthcare. But we are not. Despite these changes, America's healthcare system continues to decline. More people than ever before are uninsured; costs are higher than ever; there is more administrative inefficiency; and quality is erratic. Our healthcare system may have been even more of a mess without these changes. But these minimal changes may also have preempted comprehensive reform that could have made a real difference.

Incremental reform proposals, however well intentioned, are doomed to disappoint. All piecemeal reforms are palliative. Most of these repair attempts can't solve the single problem they are aimed at; none attempts universal coverage or keeping the cost of healthcare inflation down. Incremental reforms, especially those at the state level, are incapable of changing aspects of the deeply rooted architecture of the current system (such as the tax deduction for health insurance or Medicare's way of paying doctors and hospitals) that inhibit efficiency, quality, and cost control. Because these incremental repair attempts are directed at only a single piece of the complex system, their desired effects are largely offset by negative reactions in other parts of the system. It's like pushing on a water balloon: Here, too, we see that pressing on one side makes it bulge out somewhere else. Propping up one part of our disintegrating healthcare system would risk causing even more strain and deeper problems. Covering more people and improving quality under the current system would be costly. And without centralized government action, some unanimously agreed-upon reforms would take years to implement.

Expanding Coverage

As human beings, we instinctively react when a child is in danger. This is certainly true with American healthcare proposals as well. We often hear about proposals to cover the nearly 9 million uninsured American children. Offering health coverage for children is comparatively cheap. Fairly comprehensive coverage costs about $1,000 per child per year.

Yet a phenomenon economists call *crowding out* makes it unfeasible to cover all children without first having a plan in place for comprehensive reform. Before SCHIP was enacted in 1997, employers covered 44.9 million children, Medicaid covered 14.7 million, and just under 11 million were uninsured. By 2007, there were 3 million more children in the country. Employer coverage had dropped, Medicaid and SCHIP covered 20.1 million children, and there were still about 9 million uninsured children. Despite a substantial increase in the number of children covered by Medicaid and SCHIP—nearly 6 million—the number of uninsured kids declined by only 2 million. Such is the nature of crowding out. After reviewing all the data, the Congressional Budget Office has concluded that "[t]he most reliable estimates currently available suggest that the reduction in private coverage among children is between a quarter and a half of the increase in public coverage resulting from SCHIP. In other words, for every 100 children who enroll as a result of SCHIP, there is a corresponding reduction in private coverage of between 25 and 50 children."

As Columbia University health economist Janet Currie explained, in the 1980s Medicaid was expanded by increasing income eligibility, while the percentage of American children without insurance coverage stayed remarkably constant. Currie's research indicates that "private health insurance coverage has fallen by the same amount that public insurance coverage has risen." Other economists have come up with slightly different estimates about the exact numbers, but they essentially agree that crowding out causes a reduction in the number of people covered by private health insurance as public coverage rises, making the overall numbers of uninsured relatively static.

Crowding out occurs when businesses and individuals look for the most economical ways to obtain healthcare coverage. Imagine you are an employer straining under rising healthcare costs, always looking for ways to economize. If the government suddenly offers insurance coverage for all children, would you consider cutting family coverage for your workers? Or would you continue coverage for existing employees but not offer it to new hires? Many workers, especially low-wage workers, might welcome this approach, which would result in a wage increase. Some might voluntarily withdraw their children from employer-based programs to save on the premium costs and enroll them in a government program.

When we consider proposals to cover today's 9 million uninsured children by expanding Medicaid and SCHIP, we can expect that crowding out will thwart efforts to substantially reduce the numbers of uninsured youngsters. If Medicaid and SCHIP were to extend coverage for all children, far more than 9 million children would have to be enrolled in the end, making the government's cost substantially higher.

Even if all American children were covered, 38 million citizens—70 percent of whom are working full time or are in families with a full-time worker—would still remain uninsured. Nor would covering all children do anything to achieve other essential goals of comprehensive reform. If it didn't reduce administrative waste, control costs, and improve quality, achieving universal coverage would ultimately result in a deplorable, bankrupted healthcare system for America.

Cost Control

One commonly cited complaint about the current healthcare system is that patients demand expensive but marginally beneficial interventions because they do not know what medical services cost. Accordingly, some experts advocate for economic incentives that will alter patients' demands for healthcare services. If patients had "more skin in the game," they might use fewer services and adopt healthier lifestyles, such as smoking less, eating more nutritious foods, and exercising more frequently. Some experts have proposed *consumer-directed healthcare* as a financial motivation to encourage more frugal use of healthcare services. This provision usually includes mechanisms to protect people from the large costs of a medical catastrophe, such as cancer or a stroke. A favored model is health savings accounts, or HSAs.

With HSAs, people receive favorable tax treatment on the money they deposit to cover routine health services. These individuals draw on their health savings accounts to pay for healthcare services. Most HSAs also include a provision for major health problems: If a family's healthcare bills exceed a limit, usually about $5,000 in one year, catastrophic insurance kicks in to cover the subsequent healthcare costs.

Theoretically, because people with HSAs are responsible for paying the first $5,000, they should use their money more prudently. They would refrain from seeing a physician for every virus or going to the emergency room for every headache. Moreover, given more price-conscious patients, physicians and hospitals would have to compete to keep their prices low.

Doubtless, healthcare insurance insulates people from the costs of care. There is no question that paying cash for healthcare certainly would make people seek less medical care. But whether they would make medically appropriate choices—cutting down on marginal or wasteful medical care and going to the doctor only for truly necessary services—is highly doubtful. After all, most patients are neither physicians nor nurses. They are hard-pressed to tell whether a black spot on the skin is a cancer or a benign mole, or whether a stomachache is caused by a gallstone, a parasite infection, or a passing virus. Most of us cannot determine the healthcare interventions we truly need. We consult our physicians to find out why we are sick and what we need to do to get better. Conducted in the 1970s and 1980s, RAND's Health Insurance Experiment showed that people who had to pay more of their own healthcare bills use fewer healthcare services. But the study also showed that they cut down on both unnecessary and *necessary* care. When we are responsible for our own healthcare costs, most of us are likely to cut back on preventive screening and interventions, such as mammograms and vaccines. The benefits of these tests and treatments accrue only years down the line, so if we don't feel sick, it's easy for most of us to rationalize postponing tests to save money.

In 1990, before Medicare paid for mammograms, 47.7 percent of Medicare-eligible women scheduled mammograms each year. When Medicare later covered mammograms, 63.3 percent of the eligible women did. Putting off preventive screening tests or visits to the doctor for what seem like minor complaints might save some money today but will make costs rise tomorrow. It is certainly less expensive—not to mention less traumatic and painful—to nip a tumor in the bud than to treat an advanced case of cancer.

Consumer-directed healthcare plans, such as HSAs, may reduce employers' insurance costs by discouraging people from seeking unnecessary care, but this outcome does not translate into a major impact on overall healthcare expenditures. Almost 60 percent of all healthcare costs result from treating the 5 percent of all patients who are truly sick, not the hypochondriacs who want to see their doctors too often. These 5 percent of patients use up their deductibles with a single hospitalization or with a few physician visits, tests, and medications. However, if such patients had HSAs backed by catastrophic insurance, they would pay only $5,000, and the rest of the medical care they needed during the year would be essentially free. The 1.4 million people diagnosed with cancer each year, the 1.2 million who develop heart disease, the 700,000 who have strokes, and many others with chronic diseases would have no incentive to be judicious in choosing medical tests and treatments if, after their $5,000 deductible, all their medical bills were covered by catastrophic insurance. Even healthy individuals can manipulate a consumer-directed healthcare system, or any other health policy or plan that employs a large deductible: People often postpone elective tests or expensive colonoscopies to the next calendar year, when their deductible has been exceeded and such tests will be covered by insurance.

HSAs would, moreover, offer the wrong incentives for drug companies and medical-device manufacturers. If all medical costs beyond the deductible were covered by insurance, drug and device manufacturers would have an incentive to concentrate their research and development on the *most* expensive potential products. It is true that people might resist paying out-of-pocket for a low-cost product that was not covered by insurance, but an expensive drug or device would likely be required after the catastrophic coverage had already kicked in. Consequently, the cost of the product would be covered by insurance. Making consumers cost conscious would not affect use of these expensive products. Over time, this sort of system promotes expensive technologies, driving high healthcare inflation long into the future.

It is clear that HSAs cannot restrain healthcare inflation. Consumer-directed healthcare does not expand healthcare coverage to include more Americans, either. And these medical savings accounts might actually do more to *reduce* healthcare quality than to increase it if people postpone essential preventive measures and skip effective medications for chronic diseases. HSAs represent another well-intentioned way to repair just *one* problem—a way that fails to improve, and may actually worsen, the system as a whole.

Quality

Americans hear a lot these days about the promise of improved information technology for our healthcare system. In particular, the adoption of electronic medical records (EMRs) and computerized physician order entry represent widely endorsed, incremental changes that can improve both quality and efficiency. Experts agree that computerized drug orders by hospital physicians could reduce harmful drug-to-drug interactions and minimize the possibility of administering the wrong drug to the wrong patient.

One recent study at Harvard Medical School showed that, with the right technology, medication errors fell 95 percent. And a comprehensive study by RAND suggests that installing a computerized drug ordering system in every American hospital could eliminate 200,000 adverse drug events each year and save $1 billion. Adopting these automated systems in physician offices not only could eliminate 2 million adverse drug reactions annually, saving $3.5 billion, but also effectively remind doctors to order preventive tests and treatments, such as mammograms and vaccines, thereby saving both lives and costs. For example, according to a RAND study, about 20,000 deaths could be avoided each year if pneumonia vaccines were administered to all eligible patients. RAND also estimates that if electronic medical records were widely used for management of chronic diseases, the number of hospital stays for diabetes, heart disease, emphysema, and asthma would be reduced by 4 million per year, while 28 million lost workdays would be recovered, generating an annual savings of nearly $30 billion. Real-time data on the nature of physicians' interventions and patient outcomes could help target services better. Mundane transcription costs would decline while nurse productivity would increase.

The productivity gains realized by the adoption of information technology (IT) in other industries have been remarkable. The telecommunications industry has achieved productivity gains of 8 percent per year from the implementation of IT alone. Gains in retail have been smaller, but the industry has experienced a respectable 2–3 percent savings per year from IT-linked productivity increases. RAND estimates that, if installed in 90 percent of physicians' offices and hospitals, electronic medical records could save $77 billion per year. Even if the savings were not this high, electronic medical records would undoubtedly enhance quality and improve patient tracking.

Given the obvious advantages of EMRs and the wide publicity they have received, why have incremental attempts to implement them failed? Currently only 13–24 percent of physician offices and 25 percent of hospitals use electronic medical records, and just 5 percent of hospitals have implemented computerized physician-order entry systems. Lack of industry-wide standards poses a major barrier. Without a single, dominant electronics or software company providing automated medical records systems and without national coordination among hospitals and physicians, no uniform set of standards or guaranteed interoperability of computer systems can exist. Doctors and hospitals are hesitant to invest in automated systems that may not enable them to share information with other providers, nor do they want to pay for systems that may become obsolete if a different product gains wider market acceptance.

High initial capital investment requirements have also impeded adoption of electronic medical records. The initial cost of an EMR system for a medical office is about $44,000 per provider. Overtime maintenance costs, software, and hardware updates take a further financial toll. For a small physician group, especially in relatively low-paid primary-care specialties, such costs may be prohibitive. (Very few solo practitioners have electronic medical records, whereas up to half of very large physician groups do.) Moreover, learning how to use electronic medical records initially *decreases* productivity in the office or hospital; most physicians end up spending more time at work after installing computerized records systems. Technical support is another bone of contention: More than 75 percent of physicians work in offices of eight physicians or fewer and cannot afford a full-time IT expert.

Financial and technical considerations are substantial impediments for wide installation of electronic medical records, but the biggest barrier is the disconnect between who pays and who profits. Most of the benefits from the added efficiencies of EMRs go to patients and payers. Insurance companies benefit because automation drives down healthcare costs; patients get more efficient and higher-quality care, so they can enjoy more time at work, at school, or at play; and employers gain from healthy, productive workers who are on the job. It is the doctors and hospitals that lose. They have to buy, install, maintain, and educate staff to use electronic medical records systems. A four-physician primary-care group in Philadelphia that spent $140,000 to buy a system and $40,000 per year to maintain it summarized their experience as follows:

> Going live [with the new computerized medical record system] rendered everyone in the office incompetent to do their core jobs. . . . Everyone in the office simultaneously experienced pervasive anxiety and unhappiness. Waiting time for patients dramatically increased. In short, people were miserable at work. . . . A decline in productivity after implementation of an electronic health record seems inevitable [because] every patient represented a "new patient" to the electronic health record. . . . Unfortunately, most of the information we receive (such as radiology reports, consultations, and procedure codes) does not come to us in a format that the system can recognize electronically. . . .
>
> We accrue no additional revenue from any current payer for having electronic medical records. . . . None of the beneficiaries of our investment—patients, insurance companies, our specialist colleagues, health plans, our liability carrier—have directly shared in the cost of implementing an electronic health record system.

Without a lot of financial and technical support, electronic medical records will not spontaneously arise. Even though offices that have converted to electronic records admit that they would never return to paper, the start-up barriers for EMRs are significant.

Yet information technology experts predict that physicians and hospitals, too, would realize financial benefits over the long haul. Interestingly, many of these gains would be produced by what is called *up coding*, the process by which electronic medical records make it easier for physicians to receive higher fees—specifically, by showing insurers and government health plans the full complexity of their patients' medical problems. However, while up coding may eventually put more money in the physician's pocket, it does not improve the quality of care or hold down costs.

Electronic medical records represent a necessary reform, but the fragmented, fee-for-service system has greatly retarded their adoption. Physicians and hospitals may overcome the barriers and implement computerized medical records—eventually. But coordination and financing barriers abound. Without a central push coupled with strong incentives, this will be a very slow process. Hence, Butler's "minimal change" approach, which specifically rejects concerted, central government action, is actually bogging down the reforms necessary for EMRs.

In Portland, Oregon, there was a recent attempt to organize the regional health information system. Portland sought to use the Internet to share computerized information such as laboratory results, imaging, discharge summaries, and surgical reports across 1.2 million residents. Sharing this information would have required $3.4 million in operating expenses per year, and an additional $150,000 per participating hospital. Yet such a sharing system could have saved insurers and patients $17 million, and offered them improved quality. Despite such a lopsided cost/benefit ratio, the proposal has stalled, primarily because hospitals saddled with the cost were offered few incentives.

Though an essential component of a high-quality, coordinated delivery system, EMRs in every doctor's office and hospital cannot solve the other major problems of our healthcare system, including coverage (see Table 5.1).

TABLE 5.1. SUMMARY OF INCREMENTAL REFORM

GOALS, QUESTIONS, AND ANSWERS

1. Guaranteed Coverage

Does the proposal for a new American healthcare system guarantee healthcare coverage for all Americans—not 96 percent or 97 percent, but 100 percent? Does the proposal guarantee a defined set of benefits that includes office and home visits, hospitalization, preventive screening tests, prescription drugs, some dental care, mental-health care, and physical and occupational therapies, with no deductibles and minimal co-payments?

NO. Even by providing all children health coverage, 38 million Americans would remain uninsured.

2. Effective Cost Controls

Does the proposal improve efficiency by reducing excessive administrative costs and reducing fraud? Does the proposal eliminate multiple financing mechanisms and redundant bureaucracies? Will the proposal rein in rising costs of healthcare inflation from diffusion of technology and cost-ineffective care?

NO.

3. High-Quality, Coordinated Care

Does the reform proposal have a mechanism to reduce medical errors, hospital-acquired infections, and high-cost/low-to-no-benefit treatments? Does the proposal encourage coordinated care and innovation in delivery, while also holding providers accountable for high-quality health outcomes? Is there a process for regularly evaluating the quality of these providers?

YES AND NO. Electronic medical records may improve quality by reducing drug errors, duplication of tests, and ensuring adherence to proven therapies. But widespread adoption of electronic medical records will only occur with some coordinated stimulus by the federal government.

4. Choice

Will Americans be able to choose their health insurance plans, physicians, and hospitals? Does the proposal give citizens the freedom to purchase extra healthcare benefits beyond the standard benefits guaranteed to all?

NO.

5. Fair Funding

Does the proposal have financing in which all Americans contribute fairly?

NO.

6. Reasonable Dispute Resolution

Does the new healthcare system proposal offer a mechanism for rational dispute resolution that quickly and efficiently compensates patients who are harmed while at the same time protecting physicians from frivolous lawsuits and skyrocketing malpractice premiums?

NO.

7. Economic Revitalization

Does the proposal eliminate healthcare considerations from the purview of business, so businesses can focus on the core competencies? Will the new system guarantee total insurance portability? Will the proposal reduce labor-management conflict and permit hiring based on productivity and not fringe benefits?

NO.

The Bottom Line

Incremental repairs aimed at reducing the number of uninsured individuals, improving quality, or controlling costs may do some good, but probably not very much. They begin with very limited objectives, and none of these measures completely solves even one of the system's major problems. Indeed, we need to oppose formidable companies and organizations that espouse incremental changes rather than comprehensive reform. Private enterprise claims it can handle healthcare reform on its own through wellness programs, cost shifting, and other measures, but attempts for the last four decades by the private system, including HMOs, PPOs, and HSAs, have failed to result in significant improvements. Sometimes these changes have shown promising short-term gains, but ultimately it can be seen that the fundamental flaws of our healthcare system overwhelm both public- and private-sector band-aids.

Some organizations may believe that dealing with the devil you know is better than facing a reform you don't know. Others support incremental reform as a means of retaining their competitive advantages and their profit margins. Regardless, incremental reform is just another way of doing business as usual. And business as usual is precisely why the American healthcare system is falling apart.

CHAPTER 6

The Mistake of Mandates

Almost everyone can agree that if we were starting with a blank sheet of paper, the Guaranteed Healthcare Access Plan would be the ideal way to organize healthcare. By combining government oversight and guaranteed coverage within a private delivery system, this Plan achieves all the goals of a healthcare system in the most fair, efficient, and sustainable way. But, some experts argue, we are not starting with a blank sheet of paper. We can't get there from here. Americans with employer-provided health insurance are reluctant to embrace comprehensive change despite all its benefits. At the end of the day, many of us prefer the devil we know. We are afraid to let go of what we have in return for the promised benefits of an uncertain future system. At a meeting in Washington, DC, in 2007, Jonathan Gruber, a health economist at MIT, likened our current reluctance to do away with employer-provided insurance to the experience of being forced off a comfortable boat in the middle of a lake:

> We have this beautiful boat called employer-provided insurance, which has 147 million Americans on it. It is very nice

> because these people get to buy their cabin on the boat with pre-tax dollars. So they have these very nice rooms on the boat, and they are basically enjoying themselves. [Then someone] says, "Okay, everybody off the boat. We'll move you onto a new boat with the uninsured and Medicaid recipients, and don't worry, it'll be nice enough."

Rather than trying to move everyone to a new system, Gruber and other experts advocate *filling in the cracks* between employer-based insurance, Medicaid, and Medicare. The most common fill-in-the-cracks approaches call for a mandate. In the 1990s, *employer* mandates, which required that businesses buy insurance for their workers or pay a tax to cover them, were the preferred reform proposal. Such mandates would extend coverage to about 70 percent of the uninsured, while the rest would be covered by an expanded Medicaid. Today, most advocates of this reform favor *individual* mandates, sometimes combined with a smaller employer mandate.

In April 2006, when Massachusetts' then-Republican governor Mitt Romney and the state's Democratic legislature agreed on a healthcare plan requiring that individuals purchase healthcare insurance, the mandate approach received a huge boost. Because the Massachusetts plan garnered bipartisan support even though there was no urgent crisis, the idea of individual mandates created broad, national ripples. The major 2008 Democratic presidential candidates and numerous state governors have endorsed the idea of mandates, although Romney actually distanced himself from the idea when he unsuccessfully campaigned for the 2008 Republican presidential nomination.

Many Americans don't understand the details of mandates, or the far-reaching financial and political consequences of legislating those requirements.

Mandate Programs

Mandate programs are especially appealing because they are designed to build on the current healthcare system, while changing as little as possible to achieve *near*-universal coverage. The three fundamental elements of this type of reform are the mandate itself, an Insurance Exchange, and subsidies (see Table 6.1).

TABLE 6.1. THE ESSENTIAL ELEMENTS OF MANDATE PROGRAMS

The Mandate: All individuals and/or employers are required to purchase health insurance.

An Insurance Exchange: All people who do not receive insurance through their employers or the government—the uninsured, employees of small businesses, and self-insured people—are pooled together to make buying insurance more efficient and to obtain less expensive health insurance rates.

Subsidies: Income-linked subsidies are provided for the purchase of insurance, and eligibility requirements for Medicaid and SCHIP are expanded to include more people.

The Mandate

Just like the liability insurance required of automobile owners, the mandate for health coverage would require that everyone purchase basic health insurance. Particularly affected by the mandate would be workers who, though they have chosen not to buy health insurance offered by their employer, would be *required* to purchase coverage themselves. Americans eligible for government programs such as Medicaid or SCHIP who are not otherwise covered would be *required* to enroll. (An estimated 11 million eligible people are currently not enrolled.) And Americans who are left in the cracks between employers and government programs or who are self-employed would be *required* to purchase insurance. Citizens—or employers—who did not purchase health insurance would be penalized for not complying with the law. Like taxes, purchasing health insurance would be a requirement of citizenship.

The Insurance Exchange

Mandate plans include a provision for the government to establish an Insurance Exchange to reduce the cost of insurance premiums and make coverage more affordable. In reform proposals, this Insurance Exchange is called a "purchasing cooperative," an "alliance," or, in the case of Massachusetts, the "connector."

The idea of an Insurance Exchange originated decades ago with Alain Enthoven, a professor at the Stanford Business School. By pooling large numbers of people, the Insurance Exchange can spread underwriting and sales costs over more people. Larger numbers also reduce the risk posed by any particular sick person, and therefore the costs, of health insurance. By grouping together the currently uninsured, the self-insured, and small-business employees, the Insurance Exchange effectively mimics a large employer; by lowering costs, it makes insurance coverage more affordable.

Subsidies

Even with the Insurance Exchange's cost reductions, health insurance would remain expensive under mandates. Requiring that all citizens buy health insurance means subsidizing the costs for those who cannot afford a policy. Typically, this objective is achieved through income-linked subsidies and expansion of the income eligibility requirements for Medicaid and SCHIP enrollment. In most mandate proposals, the subsidies would be costly because the government would have to extend subsidies to more than half the population.

Under a mandate program, most Americans would remain in their cabin on Gruber's boat. This is by design. As a fill-in-the-cracks proposal, the mandate approach attempts to retain as much of the current system as possible. Workers at General Electric, Boeing, Safeway, Bank of America, and other large corporations who currently receive insurance through their employer would continue to do so. Medicare coverage would also be unchanged with the implementation of mandates.

If a mandate proposal were adopted, some employers, particularly smaller ones, might elect to drop coverage to lower their own costs, while letting their employees purchase coverage through the Insurance Exchange. This would be encouraged. (The penalty for employers who did not offer health coverage might be lower than the cost of health insurance, as it is in Massachusetts.) Americans served by the Insurance Exchange would probably have a wider range of insurance companies to choose from, but with smaller benefit packages, fewer covered services, and higher deductibles.

The 47 million uninsured and 27 million self-insured Americans would notice the biggest difference. They would be required to enroll in Medicaid or SCHIP, or to buy insurance through the Exchange. Some citizens would be pleased to have a choice of insurance plans for the first time, and the self-insured would doubtless be happy to see lower premiums. Other citizens, however, would inevitably resent being forced to buy coverage that they deemed not worth the cost.

Assessing Mandates

Both the blessing and the curse of the fill-in-the-cracks mandate approach is that it does not challenge the status quo. Mandates appeal to citizens who like their cabin on Gruber's boat and want it to remain unchanged well into the future. However, for those who are concerned about the integrity and sustainability of the healthcare system, the mandate approach offers little reassurance to calm their nerves. Indeed, even some advocates of mandates, such as Gruber, think it is not the best healthcare policy to solve the problems confronting our current system–only that it is more likely to be enacted given what we currently have.

Mandate plans have a very important virtue—the Insurance Exchange. Almost all experts agree that fragmentation of the health insurance marketplace is a fundamental problem of our current system. With each employer negotiating individual contracts, administrative costs and insurance risks are greatly increased. The pooling created by the Insurance Exchange is a necessary reform. Unfortunately, the mandate approach uses an anemic Insurance Exchange. Rather than pooling *all* people into a single Exchange, most employers and employees, as well as people receiving Medicare and Medicaid, would remain out of the Exchange under mandate plans.

Under a mandate plan, the healthcare system would retain most of its current problems but not fully achieve the goal of universal coverage. Even the plan's champions acknowledge that universal coverage would remain an aspiration rather than becoming a reality. Over time, coverage would likely erode, not expand. At the very most, with generous subsidies, mandates would be able to provide 97 percent of Americans with health coverage. While better than the current 85 percent coverage rate, it is still not 100 percent of Americans. This inherent shortfall indicates that mandate plans have some structural defects.

Typical mandate plans propose subsidizing the cost of insurance for families earning up to 300 percent of the federal poverty line. However, families earning between 300 percent and 400 percent of the poverty line (roughly $60,000 to $80,000 per year) would have difficulty complying with the mandate. Far from poor, they would receive no subsidy. Yet a family health insurance plan that currently costs more than $12,000 a year would consume 15 percent to 20 percent of their pretax income. Purchasing a comprehensive health insurance policy would leave many middle-class families without sufficient financial resources to meet their basic needs.

Massachusetts' mandate experience confirms this flaw. Just as the state was implementing its new program, authorities exempted 60,000 residents from the mandate because the cost of premiums were deemed "unaffordable." Massachusetts could have expanded the subsidies to include these families were it not for the prohibitive cost to state coffers.

Under the mandate approach, healthcare would return to business as usual: The uninsured would continue to flow into emergency rooms for everything from mild ailments to severe traumas.

More importantly, over time the number of uninsured in mandate plans is more likely to go up than down. These plans would do little or nothing to reduce high healthcare costs or curb cost increases. The current financing system and high administrative costs of employer-based healthcare and Medicaid would remain. And although the Insurance Exchange would reduce administrative costs for some small businesses and the self-insured, this savings would be partially counterbalanced by the cost of income-linked subsidies.

Income-linked subsidies sound appealing and fair because they target aid to the poor, but they are an administrative monstrosity. According to the Bureau of Labor Statistics, nearly half of all American families experience a change of income of more than 25 percent each year. If tax returns were used to award income-linked subsidies, such information would not be available until well into the following year, at which time an individual or family's financial circumstances may already have changed dramatically. And many low-income households do not file income tax returns at all. As an alternative to producing tax documents, many means-tested programs require that people provide several documents, such as pay stubs and bank statements, as proof of income. Validating this information takes an excessive amount of time and money. With most mandate proposals extending subsidies to more than half the population, administrative costs are guaranteed to rise. As Medicaid and SCHIP have shown, the cost of shuffling all this paper for eligibility determinations for a single applicant can be as much as two months of annual premiums.

The growth of healthcare expenses other than administrative costs would also continue unabated. Because it maintains the fragmented, fee-for-service delivery system, the mandate approach offers no provision for technology and outcomes assessment or any other cost-control mechanism. To keep premiums affordable and subsidies down, the government might scrimp on health benefits offered by companies in the Insurance Exchange. However, too much cutting would inevitably result in a benefits band-aid. Alternatively, to keep healthcare affordable, the government might raise the subsidies to match premium increases. But higher subsidies would strain the government, forcing tax hikes or service cuts in other programs. (Recall the explosion of tuition at state colleges and universities because of Medicaid cost increases.) Finally, to keep costs down, mandates might exempt the ever-growing proportion of the population who cannot afford the insurance premium. As the experience in Massachusetts suggests, increasing the number of "unaffordables" might be the path of least resistance. Such a course of action would fail to curb the number of uninsured citizens.

This is not just a theoretical concern. The recent rise in health insurance premiums threatens the integrity of the Massachusetts mandate. John Kingsdale, who as executive director of the Commonwealth Health Insurance Connector Authority oversees the Massachusetts mandate, recently put it this way: "We're going to be very aggressive in trying to get those [increased rates] down to single digits. If we continue with double-digit inflation, I don't think health reform is sustainable."

A particularly thorny feature of mandate proposals is the tax penalty imposed for refusing to purchase healthcare insurance. As the cost of insurance premiums rises and the value of coverage declines, citizens forced to buy policies would become understandably dissatisfied. It is inevitable that many would eventually opt to pay the penalty for not having insurance rather than buying a policy with little value.

Add to this the impact of rising healthcare costs for employers, who are required under mandate proposals to provide healthcare insurance for their employees. As the cost of premiums rises, businesses would become increasingly attracted to the option of paying a penalty rather than insuring their workers. As a result, more citizens would be eligible for the Insurance Exchange as well as government subsidies and programs. In Massachusetts, the current penalty to employers for not offering employees insurance is a mere $295 per employee per year—far less than the thousands of dollars it costs to provide company-based health insurance coverage for one employee. The difference in cost between insurance premiums and financial penalties would determine employer and individual behavior. Under mandates, the problems of uninsurance would likely persist.

Although the mandate approach aspires to near-universal coverage, it ignores other critical problems within the healthcare system. As evidenced by SCHIP, it is likely that covering the uninsured would improve primary care, preventive care, and continuity of care in the short run. But even that claim is debatable: Citizens may choose to buy *only* catastrophic healthcare policies from the Insurance Exchange and may not purchase preventive or other necessary services.

In the end, mandates would do nothing to improve the overall quality of healthcare in the United States. Without incentives for accountable and coordinated care-delivery systems, electronic medical records, best practices, preventive screening tests, and correct treatment of hypertension and high cholesterol, the mandate model would keep health outcomes as they are. In large part, mandated heath insurance succeeds in perpetuating a fragmented, fee-for-service dysfunctional mess for a delivery system.

In failing to improve administrative efficiency and healthcare inflation, and in lacking a technology assessment program as well as better quality of care, mandate proposals would require the infusion of *additional* money into the healthcare system to cover the uninsured—which, in turn, would mean higher taxes. During the 2008 Democratic presidential nomination, major candidates offered mandate-type plans, each estimating that their plan would require an infusion of $100 billion or more each year. Health policy specialists at the Center for American Progress, which also advocates a mandate plan, estimated that up to $160 billion per year would be required to cover all Americans.

Mandate plans do not exclude the possibility of having a technology and outcome assessment institute or an organization to promote patient safety, electronic medical records, or other initiatives to address cost control and quality. But at best these would be "lipstick" initiatives—put on for show rather than integrated into the structure of the financing and delivery system. The current system is replete with examples of how "added on" patches fail to achieve their goals when other parts of the system, such as financial incentives or small physician offices, undermine the reforms. Without linking technology and outcomes assessments to the standard benefits package, malpractice litigation, and health plans' payments to hospitals and physicians, mandate plans are unlikely to significantly control costs or improve quality (see Table 6.2).

TABLE 6.2. MANDATE REFORM

GOALS, QUESTIONS, AND ANSWERS

1. Guaranteed Coverage

Does the proposal for a new American healthcare system guarantee healthcare coverage for all Americans—not 96 percent or 97 percent, but 100 percent? Does the proposal guarantee a defined set of benefits that includes office and home visits, hospitalization, preventive screening tests, prescription drugs, some dental care, mental-health care, and physical and occupational therapies, with no deductibles and minimal co-payments?

YES AND NO. A mandate plan would result in substantial but not complete improvement in coverage. At best, 97 percent of Americans would be covered through employers, Medicare, Medicaid, SCHIP, and a new Insurance Exchange. However, over time the number of insured citizens would decrease as the cost of insurance premiums increased.

2. Effective Cost Controls

Does the proposal improve efficiency by reducing excessive administrative costs and reducing fraud? Does the proposal eliminate multiple financing mechanisms and redundant bureaucracies? Will the proposal rein in rising costs of healthcare inflation from diffusion of technology and cost-ineffective care?

NO. There would be no increases in efficiency for employer-based insurance, Medicare, Medicaid and SCHIP. The Insurance Exchange would increase administrative efficiency for enrolling the uninsured and the self-insured, but these gains would be partially offset by higher administrative costs for income-linked subsidies.

3. High-Quality, Coordinated Care

Does the reform proposal have a mechanism to reduce medical errors, hospital-acquired infections, and high-cost/low-to-no-benefit treatments? Does the proposal encourage coordinated care and innovation in delivery, while also holding providers accountable for high-quality health outcomes? Is there a process for regularly evaluating the quality of these providers?

NO. Mandate plans rely on the current fragmented delivery system.

4. Choice

Will Americans be able to choose their health insurance plans, physicians, and hospitals? Does the proposal give citizens the freedom to purchase extra healthcare benefits beyond the standard benefits guaranteed to all?

YES AND NO. The uninsured and the self-insured would have a greater choice of health plans through the Insurance Exchange. Americans in employer-based insurance, Medicare, Medicaid, and SCHIP would experience no change in their freedom of choice.

5. Fair Funding

Does the proposal have financing in which all Americans contribute fairly?

NO. Many proposals use a payroll tax, one of the most regressive taxes there is.

6. Reasonable Dispute Resolution

Does the new healthcare system proposal offer a mechanism for rational dispute resolution that quickly and efficiently compensates patients who are harmed while at the same time protecting physicians from frivolous lawsuits and skyrocketing malpractice premiums?

NO.

7. Economic Revitalization

Does the proposal eliminate healthcare considerations from the purview of business, so businesses can focus on the core competencies? Will the new system guarantee total insurance portability? Will the proposal reduce labor-management conflict and permit hiring based on productivity and not fringe benefits?

NO. Implementing mandates would drain at least $100 billion more from the economy each year, forcing additional taxes. If a payroll tax is used, the proposal would be a disincentive to hiring more workers.

The Bottom Line

A mandate program would ultimately fail to fulfill the seven goals of reform for a healthy healthcare system. Although it would boast decidedly broader coverage than is the case today, a mandate would not achieve true 100 percent coverage of all Americans and would not solve any of the other problems plaguing our current healthcare system—administrative inefficiencies, runaway costs, poor quality, and the malpractice mess.

CHAPTER 7

Single-Payer Plans: An Outdated Solution for Modern Medicine

Some people believe that the Guaranteed Healthcare Access Plan goes in the right direction but fails to go far enough in terms of reforming the financing system. They object to keeping *any* role for private insurance companies and health plans, considering them (alongside drug manufacturers) to be wasteful entities responsible for coming between physicians and patients, denying care to the sick, and refusing medically necessary treatments and prescriptions. (They fault drug manufacturers for capitalizing on the misfortunes of the sick.) Accordingly, they advocate a single-payer system, believing that government should have more power to reduce costs by negotiating prices with drug-makers and setting fees for doctors, hospitals, and other providers.

Single-payer is an ambiguous term because, in its literal sense, it means that only one entity would pay for healthcare. It says nothing about how the delivery system would be organized, what services would be covered, how physicians, hospitals, and other providers would arrange services, how the payments to hospitals and physicians would be made, or how other myriad details would be resolved. Yet in discussions about healthcare reform in the United States, the *single-payer* label has become associated with a very specific type of reform proposal characterized by three key elements: a centralized national health plan, reduced administrative costs, and negotiated fees and prices (see Table 7.1).

Within the single-payer model, one national health plan run by the government would pay for healthcare services for all Americans. Private insurance for services already covered by the national health plan would be absolutely prohibited. Everyone—

TABLE 7.1. THE ESSENTIAL ELEMENTS OF SINGLE-PAYER PLANS

Centralized Government Health Plan: Behind all single-payer plans is the concept of one national health plan that would provide all medical benefits. In such a scenario, private insurance companies and health plans would not be able to offer services provided by the national health plan.

Reduced Administrative Costs: Administrative costs would be reduced to 3–4 percent of total healthcare costs. This compares to overall administrative costs of 10–15 percent today for healthcare in the United States.

Negotiated Prices: The national health plan would establish a drug formulary, specify standard medical equipment, set prices (for drugs and medical equipment), and establish payment plans for physicians and hospitals (much like Medicare does today). In some proposals, the national health plan would negotiate lump-sum payments with hospitals to cover operating expenses and control capital expansion.

rich and poor alike—would receive their healthcare services from the same system.

Under a single-payer plan, administrative costs would theoretically be held at 3–4 percent, similar to those of Medicare and the Canadian health system. The high administrative costs that plague private insurers would be eliminated. And without the need to bill multiple insurance companies, doctors and hospitals would reduce their administrative costs as well.

Most single-payer proposals include a provision that would allow government to negotiate lower prices for healthcare goods and services, especially prescription drugs. (Currently, Medicare is prohibited from negotiating drug prices.) Most single-payer proposals would establish a national drug formulary and negotiate the prices of drugs and medical equipment. In the same way that Medicare does today, a national single-payer plan would set payment rates for hospitals and physicians. Some single-payer advocates further propose that the government provide hospitals with lump-sum payments for operating expenses and determine how much hospitals can spend on capital expansion projects, such as adding surgical suites. The projected savings from the proposed changes offered by the single-payer approach would be applied to covering the uninsured and providing additional healthcare services.

A variety of single-payer plans have been proposed in the United States. One is the so-called Medicare for All approach. This plan, which as its name suggests, would extend Medicare coverage to all Americans, has the advantages of familiarity, simplicity, and Medicare's positive public reputation. Many

Americans who are beneficiaries of Medicare or have relatives or friends enrolled in the program are well-versed in its policies. Achieving universal coverage through Medicare, which would require expanding the existing agency, would be relatively easy. Americans generally have a good feeling about Medicare: Its beneficiaries are among those Americans most satisfied with their healthcare. And, most important, Medicare has extremely low administrative costs (about 3–4 percent of total expenditures).

Ironically, many single-payer advocates think that Medicare for All does not go far enough. They point out that Medicare fails to negotiate lower prices for drugs or devices and allows for-profit operation of facilities like hospitals, imaging centers, and surgi-centers to deliver healthcare services. In addition, although Medicare covers a wide range of services, it does not include other services, such as dental and long-term care.

The best-known alternative to Medicare for All is the proposal by the Physicians' Working Group for Single-Payer National Health Insurance. Eager to eliminate all for-profit hospitals, surgi-centers, imaging centers, visiting-nurse companies, hospices, nursing homes, and other providers of healthcare services, this group also wants to prevent hospitals from raising their own funds to expand or add new equipment.

Assessing Single-Payer Plans

Whether we are enrolling in insurance, going to the doctor, or getting a prescription filled, under a single-payer plan each of our medical experiences would be significantly different from those we currently undergo. There would be no annual enrollment period, and no decisions about whether to choose Blue Cross/Blue Shield, Humana, United, Aetna, or Wellpoint. Americans could choose the physician they wanted without network restrictions, and the national health plan would pay for office visits, laboratory tests, X-rays, and any other medical procedure ordered by a doctor.

At the pharmacy, individuals would receive drugs approved by the national formulary. Although brand-name drugs might not be available within the plan, the cost of prescriptions would be substantially lower and paid for if not in full then in large part by the government. Individual Americans would hardly ever have to pay out-of-pocket for drugs.

With the end of employer-provided insurance, workers who had formerly received company coverage would see a significant pay increase, as health premiums become transferred into wages. Simultaneously, a national tax would be levied to pay for the single-payer plan.

A national single-payer health plan would achieve universal healthcare coverage, and savings, by significantly reducing administrative costs. By some estimates, removing insurance companies from the equation would save $70–100 billion a year. And as further estimated by McKinsey & Company, negotiating the costs of drugs down to European prices could save another $57 billion. (Overseas drug costs might increase, however, if America were to lower its drug prices, inasmuch as the inflated drug prices paid by Americans effectively subsidize those in other developed countries.) The projected total for eliminating insurance companies and negotiating drugs is more than $120 billion—not to mention the cost savings for employers, who would no longer have to spend money on human resources personnel to manage their health benefits or to engage insurance consultants. A single-payer system purportedly could save enough money to provide coverage for the uninsured without increasing the total national spending on healthcare.

Of all reforms of the financing system, single-payer plans propose the most radical one—but they retain the antiquated delivery system that Americans are saddled with today. Indeed, since such plans are afflicted by the same problems that affect Medicare, they would face significant repercussions as a result of continuing our fragmented, fee-for-service delivery system. Deceptive administrative savings, difficulty controlling costs and improving quality, and politicized decision making undermine the appeal of single-payer plans. Not merely problems of implementation, these defects are inherent in the very design of such plans.

Keeping the Fragmented, Fee-for-Service Delivery System

Although advocates of single-payer plans propose extensive changes in healthcare financing, they are remarkably conservative regarding the delivery of healthcare services. Indeed, these advocates seem almost nostalgic for the "good old days" of medicine in the early twentieth century. In the twenty-first century, when most patients have chronic conditions, coordination of care is critical to ensure high-quality, cost-effective care.

Retaining and institutionalizing the fee-for-service payment model for physicians and other health service providers, and including lump-sum payments for each individual hospital, would remove the financial incentive for integration and coordination of care across providers. Once the fee-for-service system was locked in by the financial incentives of single-payer, it would be difficult, if not impossible, to change the way care is delivered in America.

Furthermore, single-payer advocates are implacably hostile toward insurance companies and health plans—the very organizations capable of building the infrastructure and information systems needed to coordinate care. In our current system, financial incentives encourage insurers to refuse coverage for truly sick patients. The problem lies in the structure of the system—not in the actors. With proper incentives, this could be changed. Unfortunately, however, many single-payer advocates register only the administrative waste and corrupt behaviors of these organizations, rather than their potential for lasting change in a more rationally organized healthcare system.

Coordination of care does not happen spontaneously. Well-designed systemic reforms are required to provide the solid infrastructure, appropriate incentives, and integrated information that are necessary for healthcare coordination among physicians, hospitals, home healthcare agencies, pharmacies, and other providers. But single-payer proposals contain no measures for such reforms, and their plan for payment works against them.

The Cost of Administrative Savings

There is no doubt that a single-payer system would produce huge administrative savings. But low administrative costs do not necessarily translate into low healthcare costs. And, as the example of Medicare illustrates, *very* low administrative costs can result in wide-reaching fraud and abuse.

To process more than 1 billion physician visits, 40 million hospitalizations, and billions of prescriptions every year, a national single-payer health plan would require sophisticated computer technology. Developing and keeping technology up to date would incur an expensive additional administrative cost. Our government agencies are often prevented from spending money on information technology because IT requires large initial capital investments for equipment, programming, and implementation as well as continued administrative costs for maintenance.

Monitoring the quality of care delivered to patients also constitutes an administrative expense. But extensive monitoring would be impossible within a structure where administrative costs are limited to 3–4 percent. Single-payer proposals have no provisions for conducting systematic assessments to determine whether new technologies are actually beneficial, whether new surgical procedures really lead to longer lives, or whether a newly developed drug actually provides greater benefit for the same disease as a generic medication that costs a penny a pill.

Nothing would absolutely prohibit single-payer plans from spending more money on administration to improve quality, detect fraud, develop information technology, and address payment issues. Nothing, that is, but the extremely strong ideological commitment among single-payer proponents to keeping administrative expenses very, very low. Repeatedly touting the advantage of low administrative costs creates a line in the sand, and crossing it signals a betrayal of the single-payer ideology. There would be great resistance to spending significant amounts of money on "administration" in the single-payer system—whether on fraud investigations, information technology, medical technology assessment, or quality of care. Within the single-payer approach, it is easier to cut fraud investigations, quality improvement programs, and data collections.

A national single-payer plan would require five times the amount of money currently needed to support Medicare. Decisions made by this government agency would affect every American and every one of the roughly 5,000 acute-care hospitals, 850,000 physicians, 39,000 drug stores, and 8,100 home health agencies in the United States. Moreover, the single-payer plan would require annual negotiations with thousands of drug and device companies and other providers. As demonstrated on a smaller scale by Medicare, this model is a sure prescription for inflexibility, lack of innovation, and stasis. Whenever a centralized administration controls the spending of every dollar in a healthcare system, decisions are made at a snail's pace.

Low administrative costs would exacerbate the problem of inflexibility. Without a healthy administrative budget, fewer people would manage a huge, multifarious healthcare system. And with fewer experts who understand how to address problems, assess experiments, evaluate innovations, and find creative solutions, there would be significantly less capacity for improving and advancing healthcare services for all citizens.

Cost-Control Problems

By reducing administrative costs, negotiating drug prices, and bargaining with manufacturers, single-payer plans could save over $120 billion. But these short-term savings should not be confused with controlling long-term growth in costs. Efficiencies, in the form of reduced administrative waste, are one-time savings. *Controlling costs* requires reducing the increase in medical spending year after year. Single-payer plans aim to use the money saved in a more efficient financing system to extend coverage and possibly expand services. (For instance, savings might be used to provide dental care for all Americans.) But one-time savings are incapable of restraining the fundamental forces that drive healthcare inflation. Unless a mechanism to control underlying price pressures were established, savings would dry up in a matter of years, resulting in increasingly high medical costs.

One way to control costs is to constrain the "supply" part of the equation by using government muscle to limit technology.

Some single-payer plans propose determining centrally the number of MRI scanners, cardiac surgical suites, and hospitals that provide chemotherapy or radiation therapy within a given community. In the Physicians' Working Group proposal, the government would negotiate with hospitals on capital expansion and could easily limit specific facilities. But constraining the supply would generate lengthy waiting lists for tests and procedures, which in turn would stoke public resentment. It is highly dubious that Americans, especially the upper middle class, would tolerate any health system proposal that relies on limiting available medical services.

Constraining the supply would also promote gaming of the system and inequality. With restrictions on technology, patients would inevitably try to jump the queue; physicians in private practice would feel obligated to their *own* patients and help them get the services they wanted. Countries that have tried to constrain the supply have found, not surprisingly, that wealthier patients tend to be favored. In many facets of life, wealthier people have learned to come out on top in situations where there are limits. Limits on healthcare technology would offer wealthier Americans one more setting in which to use their greater resources to game the system. Studies in Canada show that despite the fact that all Canadians are legally entitled to the same services, wealthier patients have substantially better access to constrained high-tech services like MRI scanners and radiation therapy.

As an alternative to constraining supply, a single-payer plan might control inflation by lowering prices and fees. As the only organization paying most physicians, hospitals, and drug companies, the national health plan would have both the leverage and the incentive to squeeze down on payments. Lower fees would keep costs down, and with no one else to turn to, providers would have limited recourse.

Currently, our government uses this low-price approach in Medicaid and Medicare. To save money, the government occasionally rolls back hospital and physician fees. Predictably, hospital organizations and physician groups clamor about going broke and successfully lobby Congress to increase their fees. And so the seesaw goes up and down: Prices are rolled back and then later increased. Even when fees are lowered, the system does not save much money because physicians can compensate for the lower fees by ramping up volume, seeing more patients each day for shorter visits. In the absence of data on the recommended frequency of visits, it is relatively easy for doctors to effect this change. Few studies have examined whether the frequency of visits makes a difference in the outcomes of people who have suffered mild heart attacks, emphysema, diabetes, cancer, or asthma. (When Canada's national health insurance administrators kept fees low, doctors responded as predicted by raising volume.)

The British National Health Service (NHS) used to employ the cost-control model that the Physicians' Working Group promotes; it paid hospitals a fixed price for operating expenses and controlled capital expenditures to limit expansion and the purchase of new technologies. As a result, hospitals put off maintenance and cleaning and slowly began falling apart, getting filthier by the day. Starving financially, the hospitals gradually crumbled. They could not buy new equipment or adapt quickly to changes in medical practice. Eventually, even the stiff-upper-lipped British rebelled at the polls, forcing the government to reverse course and allow hospitals to make their own decisions, including the authority to raise funds or float bonds to expand or buy new technologies.

Lowering prices and fees creates conditions that cause healthcare systems to decay, while constraining supply creates inequality and deep dissatisfaction. Neither offers a sustainable approach to cost control. Yet doing nothing and watching healthcare costs rise forever are not realistic options, either.

Politicization of Decision Making

Experience tells us that every decision made within a government-administered, single-payer system would be inherently political. In the best of scenarios, a single-payer system would be run by a wise, honest, omniscient administrator. But what if the devil seized the controls?

Under a single-payer system, the entire $2 trillion healthcare bill of the United States would flow through the federal government, swelling the total federal budget by about 50 percent. Indeed, healthcare would constitute the fastest-growing sector of the federal budget.

The history of Medicare offers a sobering lesson on how events would likely play out. As we have seen, when Medicare tries to lower hospital fees or equalize payments in different parts of the country, hospitals put pressure on their representatives and senators to increase payments. Patient advocacy groups lobby Congress to have Medicare pay for specific medical technologies or treatments. Drug companies use their campaign contributions and work with patient advocacy groups to prevent a Medicare formulary and forbid price negotiations that might limit their profits. Decisions are made slowly, and few are based strictly on the merits of the available options. In a recent article in the *Journal of the American Medical Association,* Harold Luft, the director of the Institute for Health Policy Studies at the University of California, San Francisco, offered a sober summary of the likely outcome for single-payer plans:

> Medicare, which provides near-universal coverage to U.S. residents 65 years and older, is the prototypical single-payer model and routinely exhibits the problems of the model. Although permitted to arbitrarily set fees, Medicare has found it difficult to do so effectively. Across the board fee changes elicit broad based political reaction; narrowly focused changes draw sub rosa special-interest lobbying. [P]atient advocacy groups, often supported by industry and specialty societies, encourage coverage for specific services. . . . Rather than market discipline, Medicare is subject to political manipulation and bureaucratic rigidity. . . . Single-payer advocates envisioning an equitable and efficient healthcare system idealistically disregard the example of Medicare and the ethos of the U.S. political system.

Because a single-payer plan would be subject to annual appropriations and lobbying, it would be vulnerable to political lobbying. This is a problem the Guaranteed Healthcare Access Plan would avoid—specifically because it proposes an independent structure, the National Health Board, with dedicated funding and greater autonomy (see Table 7.2). For single-payer advocates preoccupied with administrative savings and eliminating insurance companies, devising the institutions necessary to efficiently and fairly operate the American healthcare system is a secondary consideration.

TABLE 7.2. SINGLE-PAYER REFORM

GOALS, QUESTIONS, AND ANSWERS

1. Guaranteed Coverage

Does the proposal for a new American healthcare system guarantee healthcare coverage for all Americans—not 96 percent or 97 percent, but 100 percent? Does the proposal guarantee a defined set of benefits that includes office and home visits, hospitalization, preventive screening tests, prescription drugs, some dental care, mental-health care, and physical and occupational therapies, with no deductibles and minimal co-payments?

YES. 100 percent of Americans would be covered under a national single-payer plan.

2. Effective Cost Controls

Does the proposal improve efficiency by reducing excessive administrative costs and reducing fraud? Does the proposal eliminate multiple financing mechanisms and redundant bureaucracies? Will the proposal rein in rising costs of healthcare inflation from diffusion of technology and cost-ineffective care?

YES AND NO. There would be a reduction of administrative waste by insurance companies and reduced prices for many excessively priced medical services, such as drugs. However, the lack of administrative capacity would leave the system open to fraud. More importantly, none of the cost-control options used in single-payer plans would work. Constraining supply would create queues. Lowering fees would create a backlash among physicians and other providers. Politicization of administrative decision making would make it difficult to control costs.

3. High-Quality, Coordinated Care

Does the reform proposal have a mechanism to reduce medical errors, hospital-acquired infections, and high-cost/low-to-no-benefit treatments? Does the proposal encourage coordinated care and innovation in delivery, while also holding providers accountable for high-quality health outcomes? Is there a process for regularly evaluating the quality of these providers?

NO. The fragmented, fee-for-service delivery system would remain in place. Difficulties with IT and other improvements would impede progress.

4. Choice

Will Americans be able to choose their health insurance plans, physicians, and hospitals? Does the proposal give citizens the freedom to purchase extra healthcare benefits beyond the standard benefits guaranteed to all?

YES. Single-payer proposals preserve the choice of physicians, hospitals, and other providers.

5. Fair Funding

Does the proposal have financing in which all Americans contribute fairly?

UNCLEAR. Fairness depends on whether a progressive taxing mechanism would be used for financing. This factor is not specified in most single-payer plans.

6. Reasonable Dispute Resolution

Does the new healthcare system proposal offer a mechanism for rational dispute resolution that quickly and efficiently compensates patients who are harmed while at the same time protecting physicians from frivolous lawsuits and skyrocketing malpractice premiums?

NO. No method for improving dispute resolution is defined in single-payer plans.

7. Economic Revitalization

Does the proposal eliminate healthcare considerations from the purview of business, so businesses can focus on the core competencies? Will the new system guarantee total insurance portability? Will the proposal reduce labor-management conflict and permit hiring based on productivity and not fringe benefits?

NO. Removing healthcare constraints from business and labor decisions would stimulate job mobility and innovation. However, tax increases to fund a single-payer system would create a drag on the economy and incomes, unless costs were controlled long-term.

The Bottom Line

Many Americans have been dreaming about a single-payer plan, wishing the United States could be more like Canada. However, while single-payer plans may offer a desirable reform of the *financing* system, they fall short when it comes to the *delivery* of healthcare. By leaving in place a fragmented twentieth-century delivery system, institutionalizing the fee-for-service payment system, and discouraging the very organizations that could coordinate and integrate care, single-payer plans would prevent the improvement of the healthcare delivery for decades.

In their zeal, single-payer advocates seem to forget how American institutions and governmental agencies actually operate. They envision superbly efficient, incorruptible bureaucracies capable of rational policy choices. Unfortunately, American governmental agencies do not spontaneously operate this way. Careful institutional design is needed. Even with well-intentioned government administrators and officials in place, increased fraud, inflexibility, and politicization of decision making would prevent single-payer plans from improving healthcare quality and controlling costs.

CHAPTER 8

Opening the Door to Comprehensive Change: Will the System Get Better? When? How?

Representative Claude Pepper was a renowned Florida Congressman who died in 1989 at the age of 89 after a decades-long career advocating for comprehensive healthcare reform. Before he entered heaven, the story goes, he had a conversation with God. Said Pepper, "I worked all my life trying to get the United States to enact some kind of universal coverage, so that all Americans could have health insurance. But even though I lived almost 90 years on earth, I died before it could happen. Please God, I have just one request—just tell me when will the United States guarantee all Americans health coverage?" God responded, "Not in my lifetime."

There is ample reason to be pessimistic about the possibility of comprehensive healthcare reform. In the 1930s, President Franklin D. Roosevelt, who had enough power to push through Social Security and the many other legislative landmarks of the

New Deal, nonetheless declined to try for universal healthcare coverage because he thought it a futile effort. In 1948, President Harry S. Truman's single-payer plan was soundly defeated. In the 1960s, President Lyndon B. Johnson, one of the greatest legislative strategists ever to hold the presidency, opted for Medicare and Medicaid rather than comprehensive universal coverage. In the early 1970s, the unlikely triumvirate of President Richard M. Nixon, Senator Edward Kennedy, and Representative Wilbur Mills (chairman of the powerful House Ways and Means Committee) was unable to enact universal coverage based on employer mandates. And in 1993–1994, President Bill Clinton's Health Security Act failed to even come to a vote in the House of Representatives or Senate.

Beyond the lessons of history, several obstacles stand in the way of reform. One is the *Rule of Satisfaction.* Although 16 percent of the American population is uninsured, 84 percent have some kind of healthcare coverage. Many of us, particularly Medicare recipients and Americans with generous private coverage, are relatively satisfied with our health insurance. Furthermore, many organizations, including health insurance companies, drug and device manufacturers, and hospital supply companies, are quite satisfied with their healthy chunk of the more than $2 trillion being spent on healthcare today. For them, any proposed comprehensive reform is fraught with possible adverse outcomes.

Another obstacle blocking the path of healthcare reform harks back to the *James Madison Rule of Government.* The American system of government was intentionally designed to preclude sweeping changes. To protect against tyranny and minimize the chances that a particular individual or group could generate wholesale changes against the will of the people, our founding fathers created a system of checks and balances. All proposed legislation must pass both houses of Congress and the president before becoming law. This is quite a gauntlet to run, and it presents manifold opportunities for special-interest groups to effectively thwart legislative initiatives. Furthermore, passing almost any bill in the Senate today requires a supermajority of 60 votes—a margin that previously pertained only to the most momentous legislation such as the Civil Rights Acts. This makes innovative legislation difficult but pandering easy.

In no small part, such a design has made the United States a land of special interests. Healthcare is no different. A comprehensive healthcare reform proposal must rise above the clamor created by competing initiatives. While some vigorously campaign for universal coverage, others focus on coverage for children, and still others want more resources or universal coverage for a particular disease, such as cancer. Some Americans want more focus on the implementation of electronic medical records, and others lobby for resources devoted to patient safety. While each of these groups may generally support comprehensive reform, their real commitment—the activity that stimulates their engagement and maintains their lobbying efforts—is to their own individual issue or cause.

Add to these *Machiavelli's Rule of Reform*. Every major reform will create winners and losers. Machiavelli advised the prince to remember that prospective losers are likely to be much more ardent, vociferous, and ferocious in their opposition to change than potential winners will be in its promotion: "There is nothing more difficult to carry out, nor more doubtful of success, nor more dangerous to handle, than to initiate a new order of things. For the reformer has enemies in all those who profit by the old order and only lukewarm defenders in all those who would profit by the new order." Losers know what they are losing, whereas winners can't know exactly what they will win since even likely projections cannot be guaranteed. (This asymmetry in the passion of winners and losers has been confirmed by the Nobel Prize–winning research of Daniel Kahneman and Amos Tversky, who found that people consistently place less value on gaining something beneficial than on retaining something they already have.)

This psychological feature is especially important for people who are uncertain about how a reform will personally affect them. Some citizens may agree that our current healthcare system is suffused with problems, and they may even worry about their own health insurance coverage, the cost of drugs, or the quality of care. Yet, the complexity of comprehensive reform makes it hard for them to be sure if their lives will be better or worse as a result of the change. With rare exceptions, most of us prefer "the devil we know" to the one we don't.

Finally, there is the *Rule of Second Best*. A majority of Americans agree that we need healthcare reform, but the presence of numerous varied proposals confounds us. There are at least four major types of reform proposals: incremental repairs, mandates, single-payer plans, and the *Guaranteed Healthcare Access Plan* advocated in this book. As is commonly said, everyone's favorite proposal is different but their second-favorite option is the same: Maintain the status quo. If agreement cannot be reached on a comprehensive reform plan, most people can agree to "do nothing" or, at the very best, to "do a little something."

Despite these obstacles, I humbly think God's words to Representative Pepper were too pessimistic. The American system does change. Just think of voting rights, civil rights, and women's rights. In each of these cases, public pressure swelled, and comprehensive change was eventually enacted for the better.

There's no question that pressure is mounting to change our healthcare system. Yearly increases in healthcare spending that consumes a greater and greater percentage of our GDP cannot continue unabated. Long before healthcare spending gobbles up 100 percent of our GDP, current rates of increases will make other institutions crumble. Costs for Medicaid will eclipse state college and university tuition funding, pricing the poor and the middle class out of education and needed training for high-paying jobs. And the cost increases of Medicare will force cuts in other federal programs, bloat the deficit, and crush future generations with debt. Meanwhile, workers' wages will be further choked by insurance premium increases.

The issue is not whether change will occur, but what kind of change and when.

As University of Michigan political scientist John Kingdon argues, major policy changes occur in the United States only when four separate factors coalesce:

1. A problem attracts widespread public and political attention.
2. Major actors agree on an available, refined proposal to solve the problem.
3. The major actor or set of actors vigorously champions the proposal.
4. A transforming event creates an "open policy window" to enact the proposal.

Kingdon's first criterion has clearly been met: Healthcare is unquestionably a major problem. The issue is receiving considerable public attention, and debates are rampant among politicians and policymakers.

When change will happen is completely unpredictable. It is impossible to know what transforming event will occur to catalyze change. Even those who claim expertise in the political process cannot accurately forecast great transformations, and are often surprised when they occur. By definition, major transforming events such as wars, depression, social unrest, and landslide election victories are unexpected. And they do not always prompt the changes we might expect; hence, when the major policy window opens for potential healthcare reform, it may at first seem totally unrelated to our healthcare crisis.

Consider the road that led to Medicare. During the 1950s, as more and more working Americans obtained health coverage through their employers, it became increasingly clear that the elderly and retired would be left out. Government assistance appeared to be the only answer. To solve the problem, a Democratic Congressman from Rhode Island, Aime Forand, introduced a bill in 1957 to provide health insurance for the elderly. From the beginning, the American Medical Association (AMA) vigorously attacked it.

In 1958, congressional hearings about healthcare for the elderly generated the consensus that the private, employer-based insurance market could not solve the problem. Two years later, in 1960, Congress enacted an incremental reform called the Kerr-Mills Act, which provided state grants to fund some medical care for poor elderly citizens and younger Americans on welfare. Interestingly, both of the 1960 presidential candidates—John F. Kennedy and Richard M. Nixon—argued that the Kerr-Mills Act failed to go far enough. After his election, President Kennedy continued to call for a more comprehensive solution to the issue of healthcare for the elderly. In the early 1960s, the problem generated congressional hearings, debates, bills, and political maneuvering. But at the end of the day, the AMA, conservative Republicans, and a few powerful Southern Democratic committee chairs succeeded in blocking passage of Medicare.

In November 1963, when Lyndon B. Johnson assumed the presidency after President Kennedy's assassination, the stage seemed set for comprehensive healthcare reform. After years of debate, Americans were showing strong public concern for the elderly and an interest in a healthcare bill modeled on Social Security and financed with a payroll tax. At that time, President Johnson was enormously powerful. His years as the Senate majority leader had given him unparalleled knowledge about how to manipulate the legislative process. To augment his power, he repeatedly called on Congress to enact the fallen president's agenda.

Yet even with a public acknowledgment of the problem, a well-defined policy to solve it, and a major player to champion the plan, healthcare reform was not enacted because, despite the national trauma of President Kennedy's assassination, a transforming political event was lacking. Then, in 1964, Johnson won the presidency by an overwhelming landslide of 16 million votes, and both the House of Representatives and the Senate elected two-to-one Democratic majorities. Almost immediately after Congress convened in January 1965, reluctant congressional leaders, particularly Wilbur Mills, began to debate healthcare reform. A short three months later, another event unexpectedly added momentum: the civil rights march in Selma, Alabama. On Sunday, March 7, 1965, a group of blacks and whites set out to march from Selma to Montgomery, the state capital. But they were met by a phalanx of state troopers on horseback wielding nightsticks and blasting tear gas. TV news crews filmed the event. Our nation was aghast.

Powerful and experienced, President Johnson recognized that the "policy window" was open for a brief moment. Talking with Wilbur Cohen, his chief negotiator on the Medicare legislation, and three congressional leaders, including House Speaker John McCormack, Majority Leader Carl Albert, and Representative Wilbur Mills, Johnson reviewed the Medicare legislation and colorfully concluded the meeting by reminding these four players of a key political lesson: the need to rush the legislation through. Johnson said:

> Now remember this. Nine out of 10 things I get in trouble on, is because they lay around. . . . It stinks, it's just like a dead cat on the door[step]. . . . You either bury that cat or get some life in it. [A bill is a dead cat], stinkin' every day. And let's get it passed before they [the AMA and other opponents] can get their letter in. . . . Four hundred million [dollars] is not going to separate us friends when it's for health, when it's for sickness, because there's a greater demand, and I know it, for this bill than for all my other program[s] put together and it will last longer. . . . [F]or God's sake, don't let the dead cat stand on your porch! Mr. Rayburn used to say they stunk and they stunk, and they stunk.

Within just a few months, President Johnson rammed the four central elements of his Great Society program through the open policy window created by the 1964 Democratic landslide and the aborted Selma march. The Medicare and Medicaid bill was passed by the key House committee on March 23. On July 30, 1965, against the recommendations of his political advisers, President Johnson traveled to Independence, Missouri, to sign the legislation creating Medicare and Medicaid, with the former President Harry S. Truman at his side. (The Voting Rights Act of 1965, the Immigration Reform Act of 1965, and the Higher Education Act of 1965 were signed within a few months.)

As Kingdon points out, change happens when the public recognizes a serious problem, the right policy emerges as a solution, a strong champion supports the policy, and a transformative event opens the policy window. Of course, this is a rare convergence of events. Today, though, many citizens accept that the organization of healthcare is a critical problem. Many people and groups are campaigning to advocate for reform. Safeway is calling for reform, and WalMart has teamed up with some unions to explore possibilities, and many business groups are looking at different reform plans. It is likely, with the recent economic downturn and the continuing increases in Medicaid costs, that state governments will become more active champions of reform.

But right now there is a cacophony. Before the champions can do their job effectively, they must coalesce around a single comprehensive reform proposal that they are all willing to fight for. That has not yet happened.

In November 1991, no one predicted that Harris Wofford's focus on healthcare would carry him to victory in Pennsylvania's special senate election and catapult healthcare into the public spotlight during the 1992 presidential race. The issue of healthcare had grown into an acknowledged public problem, and the elections of Wofford to the Senate and then Bill Clinton to the presidency had flung open the policy window. Unfortunately, the opportunity was squandered. The absence of a clear, agreed-upon policy to push through Congress in the weeks after the election deflated the momentum for overcoming all the various barriers to reform.

Many experts believe that if a healthcare bill had been introduced into the new Congress right after Clinton's inauguration, it could have been enacted. But that's not what happened. Instead, President Clinton established a large task force that worked in secrecy for months in the Old Executive Office Building next to the White House to produce a bill that ran more than 1,200 pages long. The delay and the secrecy were deadly. The coalition committed to enacting legislation dissipated while opposition forces, especially the health insurance industry, coalesced and campaigned against the proposal—a scenario much like the one Machiavelli predicted. And right after the unveiling of the Clinton healthcare plan in September 1993, the healthcare debate was delayed again, preempted by the need to enact the North American Free Trade Agreement (NAFTA). With that, the policy window slammed shut. As President Johnson might have said, the dead cat was on the doorstep too long.

Given the unpredictability of when a transformative moment will occur, and the fact that the window for major change is open so briefly, developing and refining the right healthcare policy are the highest priorities we face today. As Kingdon emphasizes:

> When a window opens, when officials are receptive to a new idea, the opportunity must be seized before the window closes. People who wish to have their ideas considered cannot wait to develop ideas, orientations, and proposals until the opportunity arises. At that point, they are too late. A long period of discussion, research,

> writing, deliberation, and softening up is needed well in advance of the policy-making opportunity in order to be ready to take advantage of it when it (sometimes unpredictably) presents itself.

During the process of designing a new healthcare system for America, it is easy to descend into the minutiae. Everyone in America has a different idea about what should or should not be included. When a bill is introduced, considered in congressional committees and backrooms, everyone weighs in. Patients, advocates for the poor, the American Association for Retired Persons, hospitals, insurance companies, nursing organizations, physician associations, drug and device companies, state governments, community health centers, businesses that purchase insurance, businesses that don't purchase insurance, politicians, and everyone else will all have opinions about what is absolutely required and what must be categorically excluded from healthcare legislation.

With hundreds of billions of dollars at stake in any healthcare reform initiative, the internecine jostling and infighting will become intense. Crafting a bill will require countless policy wonks to evaluate the specific effects of any policy on taxation, risk adjustment, technology, doctors' fees, malpractice, benefit packages, co-payments, conflicts with other laws and regulations, the phasing in and phasing out of programs, and a multitude of other details. Inevitably, negotiations, compromise, horse-trading, sweet-talking, strong-arming, manipulation, and all the other ploys of honest and dishonest people trying to get their way will ensue.

But in considering how to reform the current healthcare mess, Americans need to avoid the policy weeds. Focusing on details will only distract and create tangles and traps. Instead, citizens must concentrate on the pillars that build a strong foundation for reform: the non-negotiables. For now, and for the prospect of future negotiation over a comprehensive health-care bill, the focus must remain on the essentials.

I have argued that America needs comprehensive reform to create a sustainable healthcare system and have proposed seven essential elements of that reform. All reform efforts should be evaluated by whether they include not one, but all, of these elements. If any proposal fails to include any one of them, it simply cannot succeed in creating a sustainable healthcare system. And when the time for hard bargaining comes, healthcare advocates must remember that these elements form the bottom line and make sure that any bill that passes contains them all:

1. *100 percent guaranteed healthcare coverage* for all Americans, regardless of health status, with a standard set of benefits;
2. *Effective cost controls* that reduce administrative overhead and rein in the rising costs of healthcare inflation through an Institute of Technology and Outcomes Assessment;
3. *High-quality, coordinated care* with government oversight that fosters the infrastructure, information systems, and financial incentives for high-quality health outcomes, and that holds providers accountable to achieve them;

4. *Choice* of health insurance plans, doctors, and hospitals, as well as the option to purchase additional healthcare benefits;
5. *Fair funding* that requires all Americans to contribute their fair share to funding the healthcare system;
6. *Reasonable dispute resolution* to replace the current malpractice system; and
7. *Economic revitalization* that results from eliminating health insurance from the purview of business.

Our current challenge is to further refine and test this list of essentials. We must also broadcast it, so that all Americans can use these criteria to judge the merits of the healthcare proposals put forward by politicians and policymakers. (See Table 8.1 for a comparative summary of the systems discussed in this book.)

When it comes to debating major policy initiatives, it is commonly said that the devil is in the details. Arguing over minutiae often becomes a way to justify delays. Those who fear change or want to protect private interests can justify obstructionism by contending that they are simply being thorough. But there's another way to look at the process. At this stage of the healthcare debate, it is more effective to realize that God is in the essentials. Once we recognize the key requirements of a sustainable healthcare proposal, the details will undoubtedly fall into place.

TABLE 8.1. COMPARATIVE SUMMARY OF HEALTHCARE SYSTEMS

REFORM NEEDS—GOALS OF REFORM AND KEY QUESTIONS

1. Guaranteed Coverage

Does the proposed plan guarantee healthcare coverage for all Americans—not 96 percent or 97 percent but 100 percent of them? Does the proposed plan guarantee a defined set of benefits that includes office and home visits, hospitalization, preventive screening tests, prescription drugs, some dental care, mental-health care, and physical and occupational therapies with no deductibles and minimal co-payments?

Guaranteed Healthcare Access

YES. Under this plan, all Americans would receive coverage through a health certificate that provides the same benefits that members of Congress currently receive.

Incremental Reform

NO. Incremental reform would permit some expansion of coverage, primarily through expansion of SCHIP or Medicaid, but most uninsured Americans would remain uninsured.

Mandates

NO. Mandates would permit coverage of 97 percent of Americans; however, some would not buy coverage, and others would still find it unaffordable and be exempted.

Single-Payer

YES. All Americans would receive coverage through Medicare or a single National Health Plan.

2. Effective Cost Controls

Does the proposed plan improve efficiency by reducing administrative costs and reducing fraud? Does the proposed plan eliminate multiple financing mechanisms and redundant bureaucracies? Will the proposed plan rein in rising healthcare inflation resulting from diffusion of technology and cost-ineffective care?

Guaranteed Healthcare Access

YES. This plan would improve efficiency by reducing insurance administrative costs from underwriting, sales, and marketing; eliminate state spending on income eligibility; and eliminates employers' administrative oversight costs for overseeing of health insurance. Through the dedicated VAT, benefits would be tied to revenue. (Increases in benefits would require increases in taxes.) The Institute of Technology and Outcomes Assessment would permit evaluation of new technologies for use.

Incremental Reform

NO. Incremental reform would rely on the current system without any reductions in administrative costs and without implementing cost-control mechanisms.

Mandates

NO. Mandates would rely on the current system with a few reductions in administrative cost through the Insurance Exchange. Some administrative costs will increase due to processing for income-linked subsidies. There is no implementation of long-term cost-control mechanisms.

Single-Payer

YES AND NO. Single-payer systems would improve efficiency by reducing insurance administrative costs from underwriting, sales, and marketing; eliminating state spending on income eligibility; and eliminating employers' administrative costs for overseeing of health insurance. Single-payer systems would have no implementation of long-term cost-control mechanisms, other than tactics shown to fail elsewhere, such as restrictions on fees and payments to providers and negotiated drug prices.

3. High-Quality, Coordinated Care

Does the proposed plan have a mechanism to reduce the number of medical errors, hospital-acquired infections, and high-cost/low-to-no-benefit treatments? Does the proposed plan encourage coordinated care and innovation in delivery, while holding providers accountable for high-quality outcomes? Is there a process for regularly evaluating the quality of the providers?

Guaranteed Healthcare Access

YES. Such a mechanism would promote excellent care through fixed payments to care for patients, requirements to report patient outcomes and quality of care, strong financial and other incentives to develop infrastructure, information systems, and provider incentives for coordinated care. The Center for Patient Safety and Dispute Resolution would facilitate implementation of patient safety measures.

Incremental Reform

SOMEWHAT. Although incremental reform would encourage the use of electronic medical records, it would also rely on the existing fragmented, fee-for-service delivery system without any linkage to payment or other mechanisms to ensure high-quality coordinated care.

Mandates

NO. Mandates would rely on the existing fragmented, fee-for-service delivery system.

Single-Payer

NO. Single-payer systems would rely on the existing fragmented, fee-for-service delivery system.

4. Choice

Would Americans be able to choose their health insurance plans, physicians, and hospitals? Does the proposed plan give citizens the freedom to purchase extra healthcare benefits beyond the standard benefits guaranteed to all?

Guaranteed Healthcare Access

YES. Americans could choose their doctor, hospital, and insurance company. They could also choose whether to buy additional services not included among the standard benefits.

Incremental Reform

NO. Incremental reform would rely on the current system, in which most Americans have no choice of doctor, hospital, or insurance company.

Mandates

YES and NO. Some people—the self-insured, uninsured, and others in the Insurance Exchange—would have wider choices among insurance companies. But most people would remain in the current system, where their choices are limited.

Single-Payer

YES. Americans would be able to choose their doctors and hospitals but not their medications, which would be paid for through the national formulary.

5. Fair Funding

Does the proposed plan have a way of financing in which all Americans contribute fairly?

Guaranteed Healthcare Access

YES. This plan would rely on the VAT, to which all Americans would contribute based on what they spend. The average family would receive a health insurance plan worth over $11,000 while paying about $4,500.

Incremental Reform

NO. Incremental reform would rely on the current system, which, with its tax subsidies and employer-provided coverage and Medicare payroll tax, is highly regressive.

Mandates

NO. Mandates would rely on the current system, which, with its tax subsidies and employer-provided coverage and Medicare payroll tax, is highly regressive. Added money could come from a regressive payroll tax.

Single-Payer

UNCLEAR. Most single-payer systems do not specify what taxes would fund the plan.

6. Reasonable Dispute Resolution

Does the proposed plan offer a mechanism for rational resolution of claims to compensate injured patients quickly and fairly while protecting physicians from frivolous lawsuits and skyrocketing malpractice premiums?

Guaranteed Healthcare Access

YES. The Center for Patient Safety and Dispute Resolution would receive and adjudicate all complaints. Patients who are injured would be quickly and fairly compensated. Malpractice insurance would be substantially reduced and used only for those cases not resolved by the Center.

Incremental Reform

NO. No proposed change.

Mandates

NO. No proposed change.

Single-Payer

NO. No proposed change.

7. Economic Revitalization

Does the proposed plan eliminate healthcare considerations from the purview of business, so business can focus on its core competencies? Does the proposed plan guarantee total portability? Will the proposed plan reduce labor-management conflict and permit hiring decisions based on productivity not fringe benefits?

Guaranteed Healthcare Access

YES. This plan would remove responsibility for healthcare from employers, guaranteeing portability and eliminating job-lock and other sources of labor/management conflict. Cost control (see second goal) would free up resources for other economic benefits.

Incremental Reform

NO. No fundamental changes in this area would occur under incremental reform.

Mandates

NO. Mandates would leave responsibility for healthcare largely in the hands of employers. And without long-term cost control, they would result in a serious drain on the government's ability to fund the economy and other programs.

Single-Payer

YES AND NO. Single-payer systems would remove the responsibility for healthcare from employers, thereby guaranteeing portability; however, without long-term cost control, they would result in a serious drain on the government's ability to fund the economy and other programs.

FURTHER READING

CHAPTER 1: BEYOND ANECDOTES

1. American College of Physicians. "Achieving a High-Performance Health Care System with Universal Access: What the United States Can Learn from Other Countries." *The Annals of Internal Medicine.* 2008; 148(1): 55–75. Available online at http://www.annals.org/cgi/content/full/148/1/55.

2. "OECD Health Data 2007: Statistics and Indicators for 30 Countries." Available online at http://www.oecd.org/document/30/0,3343,en_2649_37407_12968734_1_1_1_37407,00.html.

3. Angus Deaton. "Income, Aging, Health and Wellbeing Around the World: Evidence from the Gallup World Poll." 2007. NBER Working Paper No. 13317. Available online at http://www.nber.org/papers/w13317.

4. Health Care Delivery. Gallup Poll. November 11–14, 2007. Available online at http://www.pollingreport.com/health3.htm.

5. Suzanne Goldenberg. "Expensive and Divisive: How America Is Losing Patience with a Failing System." *The Guardian* (UK). September 13, 2007. Available online at http://www.guardian.co.uk/usa/story/0,,2167865,00.html.

6. E. J. Emanuel. "What Cannot Be Said on Television About Health Care." *Journal of the American Medical Association.* 2007; 297(19): 2131–2133. Available online at http://jama.ama-assn.org/cgi/content/full/297/19/2131.

CHAPTER 2: THE GOALS OF REFORM

The Uninsured

1. Institute of Medicine, Board on Health Care Services, Committee on the Consequences of Uninsurance. *Care Without Coverage: Too Little, Too Late.* Washington, DC: National Academy Press, 2002.

2. J. Hadley. "Insurance Coverage, Medical Care Use, and Short-Term Health Changes Following an Unintentional Injury or the Onset of a Chronic Condition." *Journal of the American Medical Association.* 2007; 297(10):1073–1084. Available online at http://jama.ama-assn.org/cgi/content/full/297/10/1073.

Healthcare Costs

3. "Health Care Costs: A Primer. Key Information on Health Care Costs and Their Impact." Issued August 2007 by the Henry J. Kaiser Family Foundation. Available online at http://www.kff.org/insurance/upload/7670.pdf.

4. P. R. Orszag and P. Ellis. "The Challenge of Rising Health Care Costs—A View from the Congressional Budget Office." *The New England Journal of Medicine.* 2007; 357 (18):1793–1795. Available online at http://content.nejm.org/cgi/content/full/357/18/1793.

5. "2007 Annual Report of the Boards of Trustees of the Federal Hospital Insurance and Federal Supplementary Medical Insurance Trust Funds." Issued by the Boards of Trustees, Federal Hospital Insurance and Federal Supplementary Medical Insurance. Washington, DC, April 23, 2007. Available online at http://www.cms.hhs.gov/ReportsTrustFunds/downloads/tr2007.pdf.

6. "National Expenditure Data." Centers for Medicare and Medicaid Services. Available online at http://www.cms.hhs.gov/NationalHealthExpendData/02_NationalHealthAccountsHistorical.asp#TopOfPage.

Quality of Care

7. Linda T. Kohn, Janet M. Corrigan, and Molla S. Donaldson, eds. *To Err Is Human: Building a Safer Health Care System.* Institute of Medicine. Washington, DC: The National Academies Press, 2000.

8. E. A. McGlynn, S. M. Asch, J. Adams, J. Keesey, J. Hicks, A. DeCristofaro, and E. A. Kerr. "The Quality of Health Care Delivered to Adults in the United States." *The New England Journal of Medicine.* 2003; 348 (26):2635–2645. Available online at http://content.nejm.org/cgi/content/full/348/26/2635.

9. R. Mangione-Smith, A. H. DeCristofaro, C. M. Setodji, J. Keesey, D. J. Klein, J. L. Adams, M. A. Schuster, and E. A. McGlynn. "The Quality of Ambulatory Care Delivered to Children in the United States." *The New England Journal of Medicine.* 2007; 357(15): 1515–1523. Available online at http://content.nejm.org/cgi/content/full/357/15/1515.

10. E. G. Poon, J. L. Cina, W. Churchill, N. Patel, E. Featherstone, J. M. Rothschild, C. A. Keohane, A. D. Whittermore, D. W. Bates, and T. K. Gandhi. "Medication Dispensing Errors and Potential Adverse Drug Events Before and After Implementing Bar Code Technology in the Pharmacy." *The Annals of Internal Medicine.* 2006; 154(6):426–434. Available at: http://www.annals.org/cgi/content/full/143/3/222.

11. Peter Neurath. "Toyota Gives Virginia Mason Docs a Lesson in Lean." *Puget Sound Business Journal.* September 12, 2003. Available online at http://www.bizjournals.com/seattle/stories/2003/09/15/newscolumn1.html.

Fair Financing

12. J. Sheils and R. Haught. "The Cost of Tax-Exempt Health Benefits in 2004." *Health Affairs.* February 25, 2004; W4; 106–112. Available online at http://content.healthaffairs.org/cgi/content/full/hlthaff.w4.106v1/DC1.

Malpractice

13. D. M. Studdert, M. M. Mello, W. M. Sage, C. M. DesRoches, J. Peugh, K. Zapert, and T. A. Brennan. "Defensive Medicine Among High-Risk Specialist Physicians in a Volatile Malpractice Environment." *Journal of the American Medical Association.* 2005; 293 (21):2609–2617. Available online at http://jama.ama-assn.org/cgi/content/full/293/21/2609.

14. D. Dranove and A. Gron. "Effects of the Malpractice Crisis on Access to and Incidence of High-Risk Procedures: Evidence from Florida." *Health Affairs.* 2005; 24(3): 802–810. Available online at http://content.healthaffairs.org/cgi/content/full/24/3/802.

15. K. Baicker, E. S. Fisher, and A. Chandra. “Malpractice Liability Costs and the Practice of Medicine in the Medicare Program.” *Health Affairs*. 2007; 26(3): 841–852. Available online at http://content.healthaffairs.org/cgi/content/full/26/3/841.

CHAPTER 3: HISTORY AND HAVOC: DIAGNOSIS OF THE PROBLEM

Employer-Based Health Insurance

1. D. Blumenthal. “Employer-Sponsored Health Insurance in the United States—Origins and Implications.” *The New England Journal of Medicine.* 2006; 355(1): 82–88. Available online at https://content.nejm.org/cgi/content/full/355/1/82.

2. A. C. Enthoven and V. R. Fuchs. “Employment-Based Health Insurance: Past, Present, and Future.” *Health Affairs*. 2006; 25(6): 1538–1547. Available online at http://content.healthaffairs.org/cgi/content/full/25/6/1538.

3. R. S. Galvin and S. Delbanco. “Between a Rock and a Hard Place: Understanding the Employer Mind-Set.” *Health Affairs*. 2006; 25(6): 1548–1555. Available online at http://content.healthaffairs.org/cgi/content/full/25/6/1548.

4. “Employer Health Benefits 2007 Annual Survey.” Issued 2007 by the Henry J. Kaiser Family Foundation and the Health Research and Educational Trust. Available online at http://www.kff.org/insurance/7672/index.cfm.

Medicare and Medicaid

5. “History.” Centers for Medicare and Medicaid Services. October 2007. Available online at http://www.cms.hhs.gov/History/.

6. L. G. Aronovitz. “Medicaid Fraud and Abuse: CMS’s Commitment to Helping States Safeguard Program Dollars Is Limited.” United States Government Accountability Office: Testimony before the Committee on Finance, U.S. Senate. June 28, 2005. Available online at http://www.gao.gov/new.items/d05855t.pdf.

7. Clifford J. Levy and Michael Luo. “New York Medicaid Fraud May Reach into Billions.” *The New York Times*. July 18, 2005. Available online

at http://www.nytimes.com/2005/07/18/nyregion/18medicaid.html?_r=1&oref=slogin.

Quantity of Care Versus Quality of Care

8. Center for the Evaluative Clinical Sciences, Dartmouth Medical School. "The Care of Patients with Severe Chronic Illness: An Online Report on the Medicare Program by the Dartmouth Atlas Project." Lebanon, NH: 2006. Available online at http://www.dartmouthatlas.org/atlases/2006_Chronic_Care_Atlas.pdf.

9. Ira Flatow. "Are Today's Hospital Patients 'Overtreated'?" National Public Radio. October 12, 2007. Available online at http://www.npr.org/templates/story/story.php?storyId=15233303.

10. B. Starfield, L. Shi, A. Grover, and J. Macinko. "The Effects of Specialist Supply on Populations' Health: Assessing the Evidence." *Health Affairs*: 2005; Web Exclusive, March 15. Available online at http://content.healthaffairs.org/cgi/content/full/hlthaff.w5.97/DC1.

11. J. S. Skinner, D. O. Staiger, and E. S. Fisher. "Is Technological Change in Medicine Always Worth It? The Case of Acute Myocardial Infarction." *Health Affairs*. 2006; 25(2): w34–w47. Available online at http://content.healthaffairs.org/cgi/content/full/25/2/w34.

CHAPTER 4: THE GUARANTEED HEALTHCARE ACCESS PLAN: A COMPREHENSIVE CURE

1. E. J. Emanuel and V. R. Fuchs. "Health Care Vouchers—A Proposal for Universal Coverage." *The New England Journal of Medicine*. 2005; 352(12):1255–1260. Available online at http://content.nejm.org/cgi/content/full/352/12/1255.

2. E. J. Emanuel and V. R. Fuchs. "A Comprehensive Cure: Universal Health Care Vouchers." Hamilton Project Discussion Paper, The Brookings Institution. July 2007. Available online at http://www.brookings.edu/papers/2007/~/media/Files/rc/papers/2007/07useconomics_emanuel/200707emanuel_fuchs.pdf.

3. E. J. Emanuel and V. R. Fuchs. "Solved! It Covers Everyone. It Cuts Costs. It Can Get Through Congress. Why Universal Health Care Vouchers Are the Next Big Idea." *Washington Monthly*. June 2005.

4. E. J. Emanuel and V. R. Fuchs. "How to Cure U.S. Health Care." *Fortune*. November 13, 2006:78.

5. E. J. Emanuel, V. R. Fuchs, and A. M. Garber. "Essential Elements of a Technology and Outcomes Assessment Initiative." *Journal of the American Medical Association*. 2007; 298(11): 1323–1325. Available online at http://jama.ama-assn.org/cgi/content/full/298/11/1323.

6. V. R. Fuchs and E. J. Emanuel. "Health Care Reform: Why? What? When?" *Health Affairs* 2005; 24(6):1399–1414. Available online at http://content.healthaffairs.org/cgi/content/full/24/6/1399.

7. Ezekiel J. Emanuel and Victor R. Fuchs, "Vouchsafe: A New Healthcare Plan." *The New Republic*. February 19, 2007; 236(8/9): 14–15. Available online at http://web.ebscohost.com/ehost/detail?vid=3&hid=21&sid=3d3fc5c4-fc28–4ead-b4f2-aa27e3479566%40SRCSM2.

Costs and Financing

8. E. J. Emanuel and V. R. Fuchs. "Who Really Pays for Health Care? The Myth of Shared Responsibility." *Journal of the American Medical Association*. 2008; 299(9): 1057–1059. Available online at http://jama.ama-assn.org/cgi/content/full/299/9/1057.

9. "Blue Cross and Blue Shield Service Benefit Plan: A Fee-for-Service Plan (Standard and Basic Option) with a Preferred Provider Organization." Federal Employees Health Benefits Program. United States Office of Personnel Management. Available online at https://www.opm.gov/insure/08/brochures/pdf/71–005.pdf.

10. "Value-Added Tax (VAT)." *Encyclopedia Britannica*. 2008. Encyclopedia Britannica Online. February 12, 2008. Available online at http://www.britannica.com/eb/article–9074747.

11. Benjamin J. Krohmal and Ezekiel J. Emanuel. "Access and Ability to Pay: The Ethics of a Tiered Health Care System." *The Archives of Internal Medicine*. 2007; 167(5):433–437. Available online at http://archinte.ama-assn.org/cgi/content/full/167/5/433.

CHAPTER 5: BAND-AIDS ARE NOT ENOUGH

Opposition to Comprehensive Reform

1. K. E. Thorpe. "Protecting the Uninsured." *The New England Journal of Medicine*. 2004; 351(15):1479–1481. Available online at

http://content.nejm.org/cgi/content/full/351/15/1479.

2. Stuart M. Butler. "Evolving Beyond Traditional Employer-Sponsored Health Insurance." The Hamilton Project. The Brookings Institution. May 2007. Available online at http://www3.brookings.edu/es/hamilton/200705butler.pdf.

3. Lauren Phillips. "Health Experts Discuss Ways to Achieve Universal Health Coverage." *Commonwealth Fund: Washington Health Policy Week in Review*. July 23, 2007. Longwoods Publishing. Available online at http://www.longwoods.com/product.php?productid=19052&page=10.

Extending Children's Coverage

4. Janet Currie. "Appendix D: What Can We Learn About Child Care Policy from Public Investments in Children's Health?" *The Economic Rationale for Investing in Children: A Focus on Child Care. Human Services Policy*. December 2001. Available online at http://aspe.hhs.gov/hsp/cc-rationale02/appendixD.htm.

5. Congressional Budget Office. "The State Children's Health Insurance Program: Summary." May 2007. Available online at http://www.cbo.gov/ftpdoc.cfm?index=8092&type=0&sequence=1#42.

Health-Savings Accounts and Consumer-Directed Healthcare

6. RAND Corporation. "The Health Insurance Experiment: A Classic RAND Study Speaks to the Current Health Care Reform Debate." 2006. Available online at http://www.rand.org/pubs/research_briefs/RB9174/index1.html.

7. P. B. Bach. "Cost Sharing for Health Care—Whose Skin? Which Game?" *The New England Journal of Medicine.* 2008; 358(4):411–413. Available online at http://content.nejm.org/cgi/content/full/358/4/411.

Electronic Medical Records

8. R. Hillestad, J. Bigelow, A. Bower, F. Girosi, R. Meili, R. Scoville, and R. Taylor. "Can Electronic Medical Record Systems Transform Health Care? Potential Health Benefits, Savings, and Costs." *Health*

Affairs. 2005; 24(5): 1103–1117. Available online at http://content.healthaffairs.org/cgi/content/full/24/5/1103.

9. R. J. Baron, E. L. Fabens, M. Schiffman, and E. Wolf. "Electronic Health Records: Just Around the Corner? Or Over the Cliff?" *The Annals of Internal Medicine*. 2005; 143(3): 222–226. Available online at http://www.annals.org/cgi/content/full/143/3/222.

CHAPTER 6: THE MISTAKE OF MANDATES

Mandates in Massachusetts

1. J. Gruber. "The Massachusetts Health Care Revolution: A Local Start for Universal Coverage." *Hastings Center Report*. 2006; 36 (5): 14–19. Available online at http://econ-www.mit.edu/files/978.

2. "Find Insurance: Individuals & Families: Frequently Asked Questions." Commonwealth Care Health Insurance Program, Commonwealth Health Insurance Connector. 2008. Available online at http://www.mahealthconnector.org/portal/site/connector/menuitem.afc6a36a62ec1a50dbef6f47d7468a0c/?fiShown=default#q03.

3. K. Sack. "Massachusetts Faces a Test on Health Care." *The New York Times*. November 25, 2007. Available online at http://www.nytimes.com/2007/11/25/us/politics/25mass.html?pagewanted=prin.

4. A. Dembner. "Most Firms Comply with Health Law, But About 500 Opt to Pay Fine Instead." *The Boston Globe*. November 22, 2007. Available online at http://boston.com/news/health/articles/2007/11/22/most_firms_comply_with_health_law/.

Presidential Mandates

5. R. Montagne and J. Rovner. "Presidential Candidates Discuss Health Care Plans." National Public Radio. November 26, 2007. Available online at http://www.npr.org/templates/story/story.php?storyId=16612704.

6. "2008 Presidential Candidate Health Care Proposals: Side by Side Summary." Health08.org: The Henry J. Kaiser Foundation. 2008. Available online at http://www.health08.org/sidebyside.cfm.

Mandate Features

7. A. C. Enthoven. "Employment-Based Health Insurance Is Failing: Now What?" *Health Affairs*. May 28, 2003; W3: 237–249. Available online at http://content.healthaffairs.org/cgi/content/full/hlthaff.w3.237v1/DC1.

8. J. M. Lambrew, J. D. Podesta, and T. L. Shaw. "Change in Challenging Times: A Plan for Extending and Improving Health Coverage. *Health Affairs*. March 23, 2005; W5: 119–132. Available online at http://content.healthaffairs.org/cgi/content/full/hlthaff.w5.119/DC1.

CHAPTER 7: SINGLE-PAYER PLANS: AN OUTDATED SOLUTION FOR MODERN MEDICINE

Singler-Payer Proposals

1. "Press Release: Kennedy and Dingell Fight for Medicare for All." Senator Edward Kennedy, United States Senator for Massachusetts. April 25, 2007. Available online at http://kennedy.senate.gov/newsroom/press_release.cfm?id=B30A5C7B–35AC–4CC9–8192–1B1E50FC8356.

2. P. Stark. "Medicare for All." *The Nation*. February 6, 2006. Available online at http://www.thenation.com/doc/20060206/stark.

3. The Physicians' Working Group for Single-Payer National Health Insurance. "Proposal of the Physicians' Working Group for Single-Payer National Health Insurance." *Journal of the American Medical Association.* 2003; 290(6):798–805. Available online at http://jama.ama-assn.org/cgi/content/full/290/6/798.

Obstacles to Single-Payer Plans

4. S. Pearlstein. "Adding Up the Reasons for Expensive Health Care." *The Washington Post*. February 14, 2007; D01. Available online at http://www.washingtonpost.com/wp-dyn/content/article/2007/02/13/AR2007021301149_pf.html.

5. McKinsey Global Institute. "Accounting for the Cost of Healthcare in the United States." January 2007. Available online at http://www.mckinsey.com/mgi/rp/healthcare/accounting_cost_healthcare.asp.

6. L. L. Roos, R. Walld, J. Uhanova, and R. Bond. "Physician Visits, Hospitalizations, and Socioeconomic Status: Ambulatory Care Sensitive Conditions in a Canadian Setting." *Health Services Research.* 2005; 40 (4): 1167–1185. Available online at http://www.blackwell-synergy.com/doi/full/10.1111/j.1475–6773.2005.00407.x.

7. H. S. Luft. "Universal Health Care Coverage: A Potential Hybrid Solution." *Journal of the American Medical Association.* 2007; 297(10): 1115–1118. Available online at http://jama.ama-assn.org/cgi/content/full/297/10/1115.

CHAPTER 8: OPENING THE DOOR TO COMPREHENSIVE CHANGE: WILL THE SYSTEM GET BETTER? WHEN? HOW?

Status Quo Insurance Satisfaction

1. "Health Insurance Survey: Summary and Chartpack." The Kaiser Family Foundation. October 2004. [See page 4 regarding insured adults' satisfaction with their health plans.] Available online at http://www.kff.org/insurance/upload/2003-Health-Insurance-Survey-Summary-and-Chartpack.pdf.

Risk Aversion

2. D. Kahneman and A. Tversky. "Prospect Theory: An Analysis of Decision Under Risk." *Econometrica.* March 1979; 47(2): 263–292. Available online at http://www.jstor.org/view/00129682/di952639/95p0222r/0.

Special Interests

3. S. H. Landers and A. R. Sehgal. "Health Care Lobbying in the United States." *The American Journal of Medicine.* 2004; 116(7): 474–477.

Keys to Successful Change

4. John Kingdon. *Agendas, Alternatives, and Public Policies.* Boston: Little, Brown, 1984; 2nd ed., New York: Harper Collins, 1995.

ACKNOWLEDGMENTS

The creation of this book has been helped enormously by the valuable insights, comments, and criticisms from many people. Many thanks must go to Alan Wertheimer of the NIH Department of Bioethics, Terry Gardiner, Bill Blake, and Tanya Karwaki of Healthcarevouchers.org, and Karen Merrikin of Group Health for their helpful comments and criticisms. Thanks also to Bruce Agnew and Brydie Ragan for advice on editing the manuscript. Colleen Denny provided indispensible research assistance and editing advice. Drew Westen helped with trying to figure out how to frame certain issues. Michael Millenson read an early draft of the whole manuscript and offered brutally honest and therefore extremely helpful comments about reorganizing and reconceiving the whole effort. Of course none of these people bears responsibility for the final product as I had to synthesize their views into my own words.

I want to thank all the people at PublicAffairs, including Peter Osnos and Susan Weinberg, for agreeing to go forward with a policy wonk book. Special thanks to my editor, Morgen van Vorst, for reading the book not once, but twice, and enduring my idiosyncratic writing style, stubbornness, and other character defects. Thanks also to my agent Mort Janklow.

Finally, special thanks to Vic Fuchs without whom this book would never have come to be either in the imagining or the page. We have collaborated for nearly five years on healthcare reform. Through discussions and papers, we have refined our analysis of the system's problems and developed the reform plan delineated in Chapter 4. We are truly the odd couple. A renowned economist, Vic is precise and careful; he cares passionately about accuracy, such as the difference between wages and income. Vic turns over phrases and polishes them until they are pithy, illuminating, and eloquent. I am exuberant, with a tendency to hyperbole for effect. Yet we have come to see healthcare through the same lens and now complete each others' thoughts—mostly. This book is a synthesis and expansion of our writings over the years. We began working on it together, but uncontrollable events, especially the death of Vic's wife, Bev, have made completing it together impossible. Vic has insisted that I complete and publish this book, and that we continue our productive collaboration on papers and projects. Always the better for listening to Vic, I have proceeded. And I thank him for agreeing to write his eloquent Foreword.

ABOUT THE AUTHOR

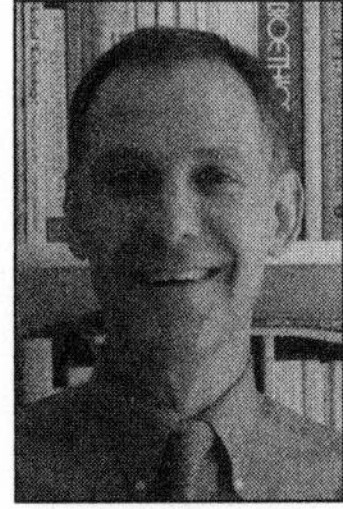

Ezekiel J. Emanuel is the Chair of the Department of Bioethics at the Clinical Center of the National Institutes of Health and a breast oncologist. A member of the National Institute of Medicine, he has been a visiting professor at the University of Pittsburgh School of Medicine, UCLA, John Hopkins Medical School, and Stanford Medical School. He lives in Evanston, Illinois.

Victor R. Fuchs is the Henry J. Kaiser Professor Emeritus at Stanford University. The author of many books, he lives in Stanford, California.

INDEX

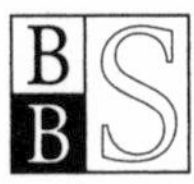

PublicAffairs is a publishing house founded in 1997. It is a tribute to the standards, values, and flair of three persons who have served as mentors to countless reporters, writers, editors, and book people of all kinds, including me.

I. F. STONE, proprietor of *I. F. Stone's Weekly*, combined a commitment to the First Amendment with entrepreneurial zeal and reporting skill and became one of the great independent journalists in American history. At the age of eighty, Izzy published *The Trial of Socrates*, which was a national bestseller. He wrote the book after he taught himself ancient Greek.

BENJAMIN C. BRADLEE was for nearly thirty years the charismatic editorial leader of *The Washington Post*. It was Ben who gave the *Post* the range and courage to pursue such historic issues as Watergate. He supported his reporters with a tenacity that made them fearless and it is no accident that so many became authors of influential, best-selling books.

ROBERT L. BERNSTEIN, the chief executive of Random House for more than a quarter century, guided one of the nation's premier publishing houses. Bob was personally responsible for many books of political dissent and argument that challenged tyranny around the globe. He is also the founder and longtime chair of Human Rights Watch, one of the most respected human rights organizations in the world.

• • •

For fifty years, the banner of Public Affairs Press was carried by its owner Morris B. Schnapper, who published Gandhi, Nasser, Toynbee, Truman, and about 1,500 other authors. In 1983, Schnapper was described by *The Washington Post* as "a redoubtable gadfly." His legacy will endure in the books to come.

Peter Osnos, *Founder and Editor-at-Large*